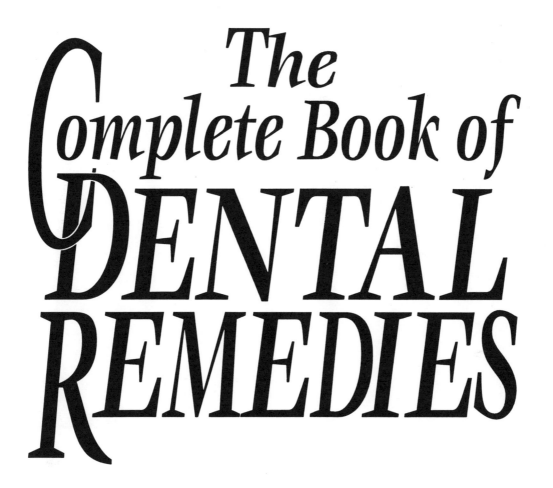

The Complete Book of DENTAL REMEDIES

Flora Parsa Stay, DDS

Avery Publishing Group
Garden City Park, New York

The medical information and procedures contained in this book are based upon the research and personal and professional experiences of the author. They are not intended as a substitute for consulting with your dentist or other health-care provider. Any attempt to diagnose and treat an illess should be done under the direction of a qualified health-care professional.

The publisher does not advocate the use of any particular health-care protocol, but believes that the information in this book should be available to the public. The publisher and author are not responsible for any adverse effects or consequences resulting from the use of any of the suggestions, preparations, or procedures discussed in this book. Should the reader have any questions regarding the appropriateness of any procedure or preparation mentioned, the author and the publisher strongly suggest consulting a qualified health-care advisor.

Cover Designers: William Gonzalez and Rudy Shur
Text Illustrator: John Wincek
Typesetter: Bonnie Freid
Illustration Layouts: Nuno Faisca
Printer: Paragon Press, Honesdale, PA

Avery Publishing Group
120 Old Broadway
Garden City Park, NY 11040
1-800-548-5757

Library of Congress Cataloging-in-Publication Data

Parsa Stay, Flora.
    The complete book of dental remedies : a guide to nutritional and
conventional dental care / Flora Parsa Stay.
        p. cm.
    Includes index.
    ISBN 0-89529-657-8
    1. Dentistry—Popular works.   2. Nutrition and dental health.
3. Teeth—Care and hygiene.   I. Title.
RK61.P26 1995
617.6—dc20   95–9682
                                                     CIP

Printed in the United States of America

10 9 8 7 6 5 4 3 2

Contents

Part Three   Dental Techniques

To my father,
Dr. Ahmad Parsa.

Preface

During more than twenty years of practicing dentistry, I have found that most people are dental illiterates. I learned that many individuals blindly follow the treatment prescribed by their dentists and ask no questions, whether or not they understand the treatment. Others are more concerned with cost, and choose the treatment that fits their pocketbooks. Of course, neither of these approaches is appropriate. Having spent many hours educating my patients on treatment choices and preventive care, I decided it was time for my patients to take some responsibility for their dental health.

I felt I could reach more people through radio and started "Dental Update" in 1985. This program was broadcast for approximately seven years in the southern California area. As I listened to people's questions and read their letters, it became apparent that the same information needed to be heard many times before it was fully comprehended. Many individuals requested written information, and I found that diagrams helped enhance their understanding. It became obvious that there was only one way to meet people's needs: provide the information in book form.

Dentistry, as a whole, is rapidly incorporating new approaches to treatment. Unfortunately, the average individual does not have access to publications specifically addressing dental care. As a dentist in private practice in Oxnard, California, who has also taught at U.C.L.A., researched and developed a toothpaste and mouthwash, and written many articles on dentistry, I felt it was time to share my knowledge through this book.

Many years of experience, research, and love have gone into this work. In an effort to help you become dental-wise, this book discusses the essentials related to dental health (the oral cavity, diet and nutrition, treatment options), various dental conditions, and the techniques for treating these conditions—both at home and in the dentist's office. Should you have additional questions, you should refer to texts involving health in general, to your dentist or other health-care practitioner, or to one of the schools listed beginning on page 203.

I look forward to writing future editions of this book in an endeavor to keep you up-to-date with scientific advances in dental treatments, supplements, and any other information that may help you to become dental-wise.

How to Use This Book

Dental care is unique. Caring for your teeth requires basic knowledge of a particular part of the body, as well as the ability to perform specific in-home techniques. A thorough reading of this book will give you the knowledge and skills needed to improve your dental health.

You will need to know the meaning of three terms used throughout the three parts of this book: *maxillofacial*, the lower half of the face; *craniomandibular*, the head and jaw; and *stomatognathic system*, the head, neck, and jaw. Part One guides you through an exploration of the stomatognathic system. Have a mirror handy to help you learn about your tongue, gums, hard and soft palates, and teeth. This part also contains information about proper nutrition and how it relates to the mouth and its supporting and surrounding structures.

In Part One, you will be introduced to alternative treatment modalities such as homeopathy (beginning on page 29) and herbal therapy (beginning on page 33). You will also learn more about the specialties of dentistry and considerations when choosing a dentist (be-ginning on page 43). Please read this section thoroughly before consulting the other parts of the book.

Dental-related problems are listed alphabetically in Part Two. First, the problem is described, and then conventional treatments that may be offered by a dentist are listed. Alternative and in-home treatments are also suggested. To help you better understand a subject, you may sometimes be referred to another part of the book. You may, for instance, be referred to Part Three, which explains effective yet simple techniques used for various dental conditions covered in Part Two.

Beginning on page 209 you will find a listing of different dental organizations that can help answer questions or provide referrals. Dental schools and universities are also listed should you decide to seek treatment or information from them.

The suggestions in this book are not for self-diagnosis or treatment. As stated earlier, my purpose is to increase your knowledge of the mouth and your awareness of treatment and prevention, so that you can keep your teeth for a lifetime.

Introduction

Americans want to become more self-sufficient in treating illness. This is evidenced by the massive number of books and magazines on health-related subjects. Unfortunately, most of these do not deal with dentistry, except for an occasional brief chapter or article. Yet more individuals suffer from dental disease than from any other form of ill-health known to human beings. According to the United States Public Health Service, 98 percent of all Americans have some form of dental disease. Considering the increasing costs of dental care and the reports on the dangers of exposure to AIDS, people don't want to be subjected to unnecessary treatment. By increasing your knowledge of the organ called the oral cavity, and taking responsibility for preventive care, you can virtually eliminate gum disease, cavities, and tooth loss.

The first step is to recognize that many factors cause ill health. Poor diet, stress, improper physical wear and tear, and poor hygiene all play a role in the origin of disease. The more you understand the role each of these plays in dental disease, the more prepared you will be to take an active part in the health and maintenance of the stomatognathic system, which includes the head, neck, and jaw (mouth).

You will be able to approach your dentist with a new attitude of self-confidence. Feelings of fear will be replaced by the realization that you are in control of your health. Fear, which is the main reason individuals shy away from dental treatment, is the result of lack of knowledge. If you have a better understanding of the problem, the treatment choices, and the options for involvement in treatment and prevention, half the battle is won. For example, in the case of a deep cavity that has caused the nerve to be exposed, you may be told to either get a root canal treatment or have the tooth pulled. In this book, you may learn that if you seek more than one opinion, you will have other options for treatment. A more conservative approach to such a problem is a special filling made of calcium hydroxide (a paste containing calcium with a high pH that helps destroy bacteria), and another material containing a combination of cloves, zinc oxide, and eugenol. Both of these materials have the ability to stimulate repair of dentin and may reverse the damage. All dentists have these products in their office under different brand names, but whether the dentist will use the materials or proceed with the root canal depends on the dentist's approach. Choosing a dentist is, therefore, a vitally important task (see pages 43 through 46).

Poor relationships with dentists is one reason that most people have a love-hate relationship with their teeth. We all realize that for a confident smile, we need our teeth to be white and healthy. However, many people hate the thought of going to the dentist and hearing the sound of the drill. The purpose of this book is to increase your knowledge of dental care to help you take an active role with your dentist, in a team approach, in maintaining health and preventing disease. If you already suffer from various forms of dental disease, you will gain increased understanding of cause, treatment, and prevention.

The importance of the mouth and its surrounding and supporting structures such as the head and neck cannot be stressed enough. The mouth is the entrance to the body. Whatever you put into your mouth becomes the building blocks of your entire body. And if you put things into your mouth other than food—fingers, paper clips, bottle caps—you can ruin the positioning and appearance of your teeth and jaws. Remember, our personality and the way we smile are enhanced or inhibited by the appearance of our teeth and gums. Furthermore, severe pain due to an imbalance of the jaw or habits such as grinding or clenching the teeth may cause unbearable stress in our lives. (Conversely, grinding the teeth may be a physical response to stress.) Vitamin or mineral deficiencies may cause gum disease.

Television advertisers want you to believe that if you use a certain toothpaste or mouthwash, all your dental problems will disappear. However, they do not mention the numerous cases reported to the Department of Public Health of poison-related deaths of children who ingested alcohol mouthwashes, or the many cases of allergies associated with the use of commercial toothpastes. Advertisers also fail to mention the continually high occurrence of dental disease in the American population. These facts and the rising costs of dental treatment are the reasons why the reading of this book is a must.

As you learn more about your teeth and gums, feel free to ask questions and to get second or third opinions. Don't feel intimidated or afraid to ask any questions. As your knowledge increases, any feelings of being a victim will be replaced by your desire to become an active participant. Don't get frustrated, but be patient with yourself. Experiment with the treatment methods explained in Part Two; over time, you will notice which methods your body responds to best. However, no one should attempt a treatment without consulting a dentist. This book, which is designed as a reference, cannot take the place of a dentist during needed treatment.

Part One

Exploring the Essentials

Introduction

Dental care is more than just brushing teeth and filling cavities. In addition to oral hygiene and the correction of damage caused by decay, dental care pertains to preventing decay, ensuring the proper position of teeth, and maintaining the health of the supporting structures—the gums and jaws. With this broader vision in mind, it becomes apparent that the overall health of the jaws, head, and neck areas—*the stomatognathic system*—is vital to dental health. Therefore, understanding the constituent parts of the stomatognathic system (gums, jaws, palate, tongue, teeth, salivary glands, etc.) is essential to our adequately caring for our own dental health and to effectively communicating with our dentists.

In Part One, we look at the various parts of the stomatognathic system. Text and illustrations are presented in order to familiarize you with the system and enable you to understand the specific topics covered in Parts Two and Three. It is essential to grasp the basics in each section of Part One before going on to the rest of the book.

The things that go into your mouth are, of course, crucial to dental health. For this reason, Part One includes a discussion of diet and nutrition, including information about the vitamins and minerals necessary to good health. Essential, too, to dental health is the selection of a dentist. On pages 43 through 46, you will find practical—perhaps even life-saving—advice on choosing a dentist. Remember, however, that your health ultimately rests in your own hands. It is important for you to learn as much as you can about dental hygiene (beginning on page 12) and about treatment options, including herbal and homeopathic medicine (pages 29 through 42). Explore the essentials and discover a million-dollar smile.

The Jaw and Oral Cavity

If the eyes are the "windows of the soul," then the mouth is the "doorway to the body." The oral cavity is situated at the end of the digestive tract and is surrounded by the lips and cheeks externally and by the gums and teeth internally. The mouth cavity is connected to the pharynx and is covered at the top by the hard and soft palates. The tongue forms the large part of the cavity's floor. The activities of these component parts require fluid, which comes from the salivary glands.

THE JAW

It is hard to believe that a backache or a pain in the legs can originate in the jaw. However, an understanding of the relationship between the muscles and bones in the jaw and the rest of the body leads to an understanding of how an imbalance in one part affects another.

The jaw bears the teeth and forms the framework of the mouth. It consists of two bones: the maxilla (upper jaw) and mandible (lower jaw). The upper part of the jaw is stationary, while the lower part is the only movable bone in the face. The position of the jaws is dependent on the relationship of the teeth to each other when the mouth is closed.

The mandible or the lower part of the jaw functions like a hinge, permitting the mouth to open and close, as shown in Figure 1.1. This hinge action is accomplished by bones and muscles located in the skull, neck, and face. There are two phases involved in opening and closing the jaw. The first phase is a simple hinge action. The second phase involves a gliding action of the joint, which helps open the jaw to its maximum. The muscles that coordinate the movements of the jaw joints origi-

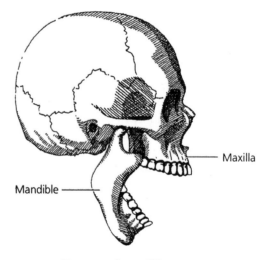

Maxilla

Mandible

The opened mandible.

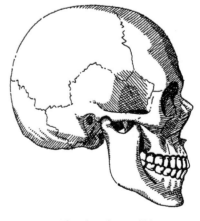

The closed mandible.

Figure 1.1. The Mandible

5

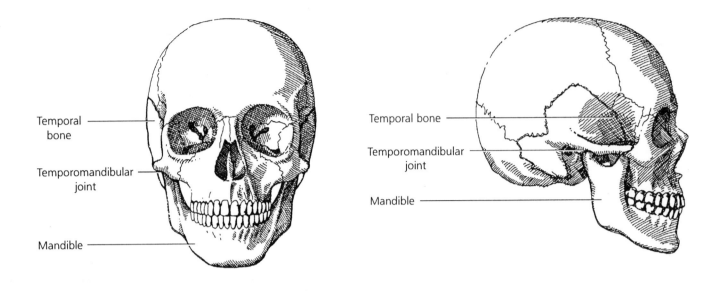

Figure 1.2. Temporal Bone and Mandible Form the Temporomandibular Joint

nate in the head, neck, and face areas. Due to the relationship of these muscles to the muscles of the shoulder and back, any imbalance in the jaw area may eventually affect the shoulder and back.

The temporal bone of the skull (the bone on the side of the head, above the ears), and the mandible fit together to form the jaw joint called the *temporomandibular joint* as shown in Figure 1.2. There are two such joints—

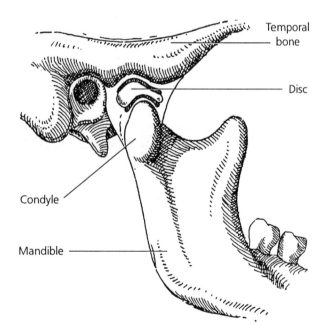

Figure 1.3. Components of the Temporomandibular Joint

one on the left side of the head and one on the right side.

Figure 1.3 shows the components of the temporomandibular joint. Each joint is surrounded by a saclike sheath called a *capsule*. This capsule contains synovial fluid, which lubricates and nourishes the joints. At each end of the lower jaw, there is a knoblike structure called a *condyle*. At the ends of bones throughout the body, condyles are attached to muscles that join the bone to nearby bones. Mounted on top of each condyle is a cushion made of cartilage and known as the *disc*. As with any joint in the body, a disc or cushion sits between the joint and its socket, which, in the case of the jaw, is located on the skull. This disc moves with the condyle and prevents it from hitting the temporal bone. When the disc is abnormally placed, the jaw may not function properly causing pain or discomfort in the head, neck, shoulder, and back area. Since the jaw joint sits right in front of the ear, any problems with this joint area may also affect the ears, eyes, and sinuses.

Opening and closing the jaw is a relatively simple movement compared with the joint movement that occurs while grinding the teeth during the act of chewing. During grinding, one jaw joint slides forward, while one slides back. This movement can be felt by placing your fingers in front of your ears while making grinding movements with your teeth. If no problems exist, this motion is performed with ease, and quietly. However, audible clicking or popping noises or pain may indicate that the joints are not functioning normally. (See TMJ in Part Two.)

6

THE TEETH

Teeth—they're not just for chewing. Our teeth perform important functions such as helping us to eat and speak, and keeping our facial muscles from sinking in. Teeth are not for opening bottles, holding nails and pins, or biting fingernails or pencils. If mistreated, teeth are subject to breakage, cavities, yellowing, and other forms of degeneration. Caring for your teeth requires that you see the mouth and teeth as important organs of your body.

Teeth are an integral and growing part of the body. The same blood supply that goes to the heart takes oxygen and nutrients to every tooth. And, as anyone who has ever had a toothache knows, the teeth are very much alive with nerves.

The better we understand the structure and development of teeth, the greater our appreciation of them will be. Practicing proper oral hygiene and maintaining good nutritional habits will help keep teeth and gums healthy. To better maintain our teeth, let's begin with a discussion of their structure and development.

Structure

The same structure can be seen in all human teeth, whether they are baby teeth (also known as deciduous or milk teeth) or permanent teeth. The care given to the baby teeth will be reflected by the adult teeth. Preven-

tive care must begin even before the first tooth appears because teeth begin to develop before they erupt. Parents are now aware, for instance, of the damage done to teeth when infants are allowed to sleep with bottles in their mouths. (See Bottle Mouth Syndrome in Part Two.)

As seen in Figure 1.4, there are three main parts of a tooth—the crown, neck, and root. When you look at a tooth, the top part, called the *crown,* is visible. The *root* is the part that is imbedded in bone and covered by the gums, unless gum disease exists. The junction between the crown and the roots is called the *neck.* The parts of a tooth are composed of various materials.

The outer surface of the tooth, the *enamel,* is a hard layer covering the crown of the tooth and the upper part of the neck. The function of enamel is to resist abrasive wear and protect the tooth from damage and pain. It is the hardest tissue of the body and is composed almost entirely (97 percent) of inorganic salts. Inorganic salts, in general, are mineral constituents of the body and play specific roles in the functions of cells.

Most of the inner bulk of the tooth is made of *dentin.* Dentin is 67 percent inorganic salts and is not as strong as enamel. Specialized cells in dentin called odontoblasts form new dentin from minerals transported by the blood. Small tubelike structures in dentin transmit pain sensations to the nerves in the *pulp,* the soft tissue containing the nerve and blood supply of the tooth. When dentin is exposed by thinning or other forms of damage to enamel, the tooth may become sensitive. When tooth decay or a cavity reaches the pulp, treatment of the nerve or loss of the tooth may be inevitable.

Cementum, a bony substance, is very thin and covers the surface of the roots. Its purpose is to attach the tooth to the jawbone and the gums. When the gums are receded, cementum is exposed, causing sensitivity to hot, cold, or pressure.

The teeth rest in a bony socket. They are attached to this bone by *collagen fibers,* fibrous tissue that forms a bridge from the cementum to the socket. The gums or *gingiva* surround the teeth and the bone.

Development

When the fetus is only five weeks old, tooth buds appear. Initially, four tooth buds, representing baby teeth, appear on each side of the upper and lower jaw. These buds undergo several changes as each layer and part of the tooth begins to form. Enamel cells form and multiply. Some of these cells begin to become specialized, forming the dentin and pulp. Next, the cells for the future crown and root begin to be arranged, and

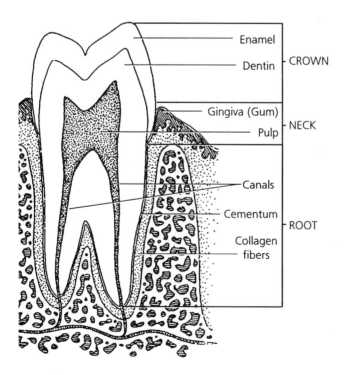

Figure 1.4. Parts of a Tooth

Enamel
Dentin   CROWN
Gingiva (Gum)
Pulp   NECK
Canals
Cementum   ROOT
Collagen fibers

layers of enamel and dentin begin to be deposited in incremental layers. The next stage is calcification or hardening of the calcium salts in the teeth, which is followed by eruption.

The process continues until approximately twenty-three weeks in utero for some teeth and up to eleven months after birth for others. Different teeth develop within this range of time; for example, front baby teeth begin to develop at five months in utero and continue until they erupt when an infant is five to seven months old. Different parts of a tooth also develop at different times. The enamel of the front baby teeth begins to develop at fourteen weeks in utero, and it is completed one and a half months after birth.

Trauma during birth, diarrhea or vomiting, feeding difficulties, rickets, and other chronic childhood diseases may cause disturbances that result in malformation of teeth. Because teeth begin to develop in utero, fetal trauma affects color or structure of teeth. Depending on when the trauma is experienced, a particular tooth or part of a tooth may be affected. For example, congenital syphilis, an infectious disease sometimes contracted during birth, will affect the teeth that are developing at that time. The front baby teeth will have notches on the edge, and the back teeth will have a pitted appearance.

Long-term treatment with the antibiotic tetracycline and excessively high amounts of fluoride in the water will cause tooth discoloration. With tetracycline, brownish bands will appear on teeth. If fluoride in excess of one part per million is ingested during the development of enamel and dentin, mottling of teeth will result. The mottling gives the teeth an opaque, chalky appearance. The severity of the condition is determined by the amount of fluoride ingested.

Eruption

There are twenty baby teeth that usually begin to appear (erupt) when a child is about six months of age. Additional teeth will then appear at the rate of about one per month. There is usually a range of plus or minus two to six months when teeth erupt and when they shed (fall out). Usually, the teeth of slender children erupt and shed earlier than the teeth of stocky children. The following table in the right column shows the approximate age at which each tooth appears.

The position of the teeth as they erupt depends on many factors. The teeth on either side and the teeth directly opposing each tooth help give guidance for proper position. If the teeth on either side or any opposing teeth are missing, a tooth may erupt incorrectly.

Age at Which Teeth Appear

Deciduous Teeth	Age (in months)	Permanent Teeth	Age (in years)
Lower central incisors	5–9	First molars	5–7
Upper central incisors	8–12	Incisors	6–8
Upper lateral incisors	10–12	Bicuspids	9–12
First molars	10–16	Second molars	11–13
Canines	16–20	Third molars	17–25
Second molars	20–30		

For example, if a bottom front tooth, which normally contacts the top front tooth, is lost, the top tooth will continue to erupt, since its opposing tooth is missing. If an adjacent tooth is lost, teeth on either side of the missing tooth will begin to shift into the space. This is why when a tooth is pulled, a replacement should be made to prevent shifting or extrusion of teeth. (See Tooth, Loss of, in Part Two.)

If baby teeth do not fall out on time, they may prevent the permanent teeth from developing properly. In the attempt to erupt, the permanent teeth may find another path in which to erupt, thus causing misalignment. Sometimes, more than the normal number of teeth erupt; these extra teeth are called *supernumerary* teeth. They may cause overcrowding and may have to be pulled. Some permanent teeth may not develop at all. In this case, the baby teeth will not fall out and should be kept as long as possible. The occurrence of too few or too many teeth tends to follow a genetic pattern, with other family members—past or present—displaying the same condition.

The position of teeth may also be altered when baby teeth are lost too early due to decay, accidents, or other causes. The teeth on either side of and opposing a lost tooth will then begin to shift and cause problems with the proper sequence of erupting new teeth. In this situation, a splint is used to prevent shifting and to keep the space open. (See Trauma to Children's Teeth in Part Two.)

Other factors affecting tooth position may involve permanent teeth that have become locked in the bone (a condition called ankylosis) and are unable to erupt. These teeth may have to be moved with surgery and braces.

Spaces between the baby teeth are normal. As the jaw grows, the baby teeth are spaced in order to accommodate their larger base. When the permanent teeth come in, they fit the larger adult jaw and fill in the spaces. Excess space may be present until a child is twelve to fourteen years old.

Types of Teeth

Eventually, there will be thirty-two permanent teeth: eight incisors, four canines, eight premolars, and twelve molars as shown in Figure 1.5. These permanent teeth will begin to appear as the baby teeth are lost—when a child is about six years old—and should all be present by the time a child is seventeen. Only the last three teeth in each half of each jaw are not replacements for baby teeth. The teeth in these positions erupt only once.

Incisors are the sharp, chisel-shaped front teeth used for cutting food. Cone-shaped *canines* or cuspids are used for tearing food. The *premolars* or bicuspids have two cusps that are used for tearing and crushing food. The *molars* are located in the back of the mouth and have several cusps that are used for grinding food. The furthest (third) set of molars in the back of the mouth are also known as wisdom teeth.

THE PALATE

As the mouth is explored, it becomes apparent how important every structure is, no matter how much we take it for granted. For example, eating would become impossible without a roof dividing the mouth from the nasal cavity. The roof of the mouth or *palate* is the horizontal structure separating the mouth and the nasal cavity. The palate is divided into two sections, as seen in Figure 1.5.

The front portion, directly behind the teeth, is the *hard palate*, which consists of bone that is covered by soft tissue. The hard palate contains some major nerves that affect the teeth. It is concave or vaulted and is the

area in which the tongue rests when the mouth is closed. Ridges contained here aid in manipulation of food during mastication (chewing) and swallowing.

The *soft palate* is located behind the hard palate and blends into the *pharynx*, the cavity behind the soft palate where the digestive and respiratory passages meet. The soft movable palate is where the gag reflex begins. On either side of the soft palate are the *tonsils*. When we eat, the soft palate automatically seals the area that connects to the nasal areas so that food does not get into the respiratory system.

The palate plays an important role in dental care and dental health. During the developmental stage of the embryo, if the palate does not fuse in the middle, a condition called cleft palate results. (See Cleft Palate and Lip in Part Two.) In this condition, an opening exists between the two parts of the palate, making eating and speaking very difficult if not impossible. Surgery or appropriate appliances can correct cleft palate. In other cases, the palate may be too narrow, and the teeth will not come together properly. In this situation, the palate is expanded with orthodontic appliances.

When dentures are worn, the palate is used for suction to support the false teeth. However, this becomes difficult when excess bone (tori) develops. Tori usually occur in the middle of the palate and may have to be surgically removed if dentures are to be worn or if the tori become irritated or painful.

With certain kinds of gum disease, tissue is taken from the palate and transplanted on the gums. Some nerves that supply the teeth originate in the palate. During difficult procedures, such as those performed during oral surgery, these nerves on the palate are anesthetized.

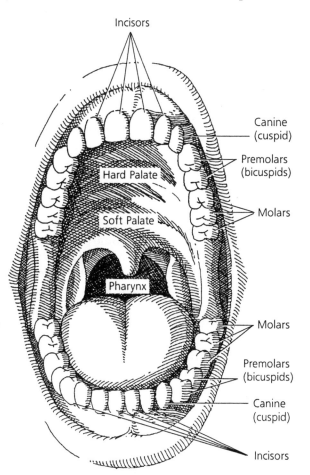

Figure 1.5 Oral Structures and Types of Teeth

Incisors
Canine (cuspid)
Premolars (bicuspids)
Hard Palate
Molars
Soft Palate
Pharynx
Molars
Premolars (bicuspids)
Canine (cuspid)
Incisors

Eating very hot or crusty foods such as pizza may damage the delicate soft tissues covering the palate. The palate also shows specific signs during illnesses such as AIDS, chicken pox, or herpes.

THE TONGUE

Forked tongue, tongue-lashing, tongue-twister. . . . Even the English language recognizes the importance of the tongue, without which we would not be able to speak, swallow, or taste. This important part of our body can even tell us, in a general way, the state of our health. And what more graphic way to express disgust than by sticking out your tongue?

The tongue is a mass of "voluntary" muscles, called intrinsic and extrinsic muscles. The *intrinsic muscles* allow the tongue to change size and shape quickly. The flexible *extrinsic muscles* allow the tongue to rapidly change position.

The bottom of the tongue is attached to the floor of the mouth. This is where the salivary glands are located. Many nerves are situated in the tongue and floor of the mouth. If a person becomes unconscious, the tongue tends to fall back into the airway, causing suffocation. It is, therefore, necessary to look in the person's mouth and clear the airway before commencing CPR (cardiopulmonary resuscitation).

The tongue is not the lively red color of the gums; rather, it has a grayish coat on the surface, caused by the specialized cells of which it is made. The muscle is covered with a mucous membrane formed into nipplelike elevations called *papillae*. Papillae roughen the tongue's surface to help it guide foods during chewing and swallowing. Papillae also contain nerves for touch sensations, and most contain taste buds. Examination of the tongue with a mirror reveals a row of v-shaped, rounded, raised areas toward the back of the tongue where the taste buds responding to bitterness are located. In front of this row are tall, thin, cone-shaped raised areas that respond to sweet, sour, or salty substances. At the sides of the tongue are taste buds that react to acidic ingredients.

The tongue has several functions. It is involved in speech, manipulation and positioning of food, tasting, and swallowing. The tongue aids chewing by crushing food against the roof of the mouth (the palate) and by rolling the food between the teeth. Swallowing is accomplished as the tongue presses the food against the palate and pushes it backward into the oropharynx (entrance into the digestive and respiratory systems). The act of chewing involves coordinated movements of certain muscles that close the mouth and raise and lower the mandible, causing the teeth to grind and crush the food. The smell and taste of food cause saliva to be secreted immediately, which helps dissolve, dilute, and lubricate chewed food. The cheeks become tense and the tongue moves the food between the teeth and backwards towards the stomach. If disease necessitates surgical removal of the tongue or if it is missing at birth due to genetic disturbances, chewing is assisted by the cheeks and the floor of the mouth.

The tongue is, of course, very active in speech. If the tongue is incorrectly attached to the floor of the mouth from birth, speech is impeded and a "lisp" develops. (See Speech Problems; and Tongue-Related Problems in Part Two.) The tongue must be placed near or against the upper front teeth to form the consonants D and T. Producing the sound made by the letter L also requires the interplay of tongue and teeth.

The Tongue as a Diagnostic Tool

The tongue's appearance is often used as an aid in the diagnosis of various diseases and conditions. We know, for instance, that during illness, some of the papillae become engorged and change color, becoming strawberry in appearance. When people have pernicious anemia, their tongues may be sore, appear beefy red, and have patchy white spots on the surface. An enlarged tongue is a sign of hypothyroidism.

According to Chinese medical science, the tongue is divided into certain sections, with each part pertaining to an organ. In this approach to the diagnosis and treatment of disease, the tip of the tongue represents the heart and lung; the central part represents the spleen and stomach; the root of the tongue represents the kidneys; and the sides of the tongue represent the liver and gall bladder. Color, texture, size, and shape of the tongue are taken into consideration as a diagnostic tool to help determine the organ to be treated.

Although self-diagnosis by using the tongue is certainly not practical, understanding what a healthy tongue looks like may give you clues about your general health. Any variation in color (too red or pale), texture (thickly coated), size (enlarged or swollen), or shape (scalloped border) may indicate an unhealthy condition.

THE SALIVARY GLANDS

Cleansing of the teeth and mouth as well as good digestion depend a great deal upon the salivary glands. A number of these glands secrete saliva into the mouth. Saliva—which contains water, salts, enzymes, and mucus—moistens and softens foods for ease in swallowing, and cleanses the teeth and mouth. The function of the salivary glands is affected by hormones produced by the pancreas, testes, ovaries, and the thyroid and pituitary glands. The nature and quantity of saliva is affected by reflexes for which the taste buds act as receptors. The presence of soft moist foods in the mouth will, for instance, stimulate less secretion of the lubricating component of saliva. Salivation or watering of the mouth can also be a conditioned reflex, as when we think about a certain food or hear the mention of a particular food.

There are a few minor salivary glands situated around the lips, inside the cheeks, in the palate, and on the tongue. There are also three major pairs of salivary glands. On each side of the face, just in front of the ears, are the *parotid glands*, the largest of the salivary glands. The duct for each parotid gland, called *Stenson's duct*, opens into the mouth from each cheek opposite the upper second molar. The parotid glands produce a clear watery secretion that functions as a cleansing, dissolv-

ing, and digestive agent. The saliva produced by the parotid gland contains a substance called *ptylin*, a salivary enzyme that breaks down starch. When a sour food such as a lemon is introduced into the mouth, it stimulates the parotid glands.

The *sublingual glands* are located in the floor of the mouth, under the tongue. The duct for these glands, called *Rivinus' duct*, opens into the mouth from the floor of the mouth directly behind the lower front teeth. The saliva secreted by this gland is thicker and ropey compared with the secretion from the parotid. Sublingual-gland secretions serve as lubricating agents; bland substances such as milk and bread stimulate its production.

The *submandibular glands* are located deeper in the floor of the mouth, under the base of the tongue and more to the side of the lower jaw. These glands secrete a mixed type of saliva that is thin at first and becomes thicker. This secretion is also used for lubricative and digestive purposes.

Hygiene Basics

Most people think brushing alone will keep teeth and gums clean and healthy. This belief is shattered when they chew a special "disclosing" tablet made of food coloring that stains plaque, the sticky, colorless film of bacteria that forms on the surfaces of teeth. When chewed, these tablets temporarily stain the areas on the teeth where—no matter how long or how many times a day you brush—plaque remains. Disclosing tablets, available at drug stores and from your dentist, provide dramatic evidence of the limitations of brushing.

How often has your dentist told you to brush more, floss more? Most people feel frustrated when they get this speech from the dentist or hygienist. Although brushing after each meal is important, it is simply not enough to maintain healthy teeth and gums.

Lack of hygiene and improper hygiene play a significant role in the development of gum disease. One study indicated that when individuals with healthy teeth and gums stopped trying to remove plaque, gum disease developed within ten to twenty-one days. If not thoroughly removed within twenty-four hours, by-products of the bacteria irritate the gums and cause inflammation (gums become red, tender, and swollen).

Not only is plaque control important in the prevention of gum disease, it is also primary in the healing process after gum and bone surgery. Studies have shown that, all else being equal, if proper hygiene is maintained after gum surgery, healthy gums are maintained over the years. Poor oral hygiene results in the repeated need for surgery and the return of gum disease.

Effective plaque control refers to the specific measures needed to prevent plaque build-up. It appears that mechanical removal of plaque is the most reliable method of controlling and preventing its build-up. A toothbrush and floss are the fundamental tools required for this mechanical removal. Several useful adjuncts to brushing and flossing include water-irrigating devices, balsa-wood wedge toothpicks, and rubber-tip stimulators. Whatever device you use, proper technique is essential. (Refer to Oral Hygiene in Part Three for more detailed information regarding these individual devices.)

Even when daily hygiene is maintained, a professional cleaning every six months by the dentist or hygienist must be included in your dental regimen. If your daily hygiene is not adequate, you will develop a build-up of tartar (hardened plaque). In this case, the dentist or hygienist will use a special instrument called a cavitron to clean your teeth. This device uses high-frequency sound vibrations in water to break up and wash away the tartar. Your dentist may even recommend more frequent cleanings, depending on the condition of your gums and bone.

Toothpastes contain mostly flavoring agents, detergents, and abrasives. Other common ingredients are listed on the following page. Do not use toothpastes that contain sparkles or added sweeteners, including saccharin or other artificial sweeteners. These chemicals are absorbed through the tissues into the blood stream. Some toothpastes that claim to remove or retard tartar may actually cause tooth sensitivity due to the harsh chemicals they contain. Baking soda is excellent for use as a toothpaste.

MOUTHWASH AND TOOTHPASTE INGREDIENTS

Ingredient	Function	Comments
Alcohol	Antiseptic, arrests the growth of bacteria. Used in commercial mouthwashes.	High doses are toxic. When used routinely, it may dry the tissues, contributing to cavities and cancer.
Aloe vera	Soothes and acts as an anti-inflammatory.	Extracted from the leaves of the aloe vera plant.
Anise	Flavors toothpastes.	Known for its ability to aid in digestion.
Carrageenan	Thickener and stabilizer in toothpastes.	A seaweed gum by-product.
Chlorhexidine	Preservative, has antiplaque and antiseptic properties. Used in mouthwashes such as Peridex.	Possible side effects include staining of teeth and alterations in taste.
Ginseng	Thought to enhance endurance, slow the aging process, protect cells from radiation damage, prevent heart disease, and increase the flow of saliva.	Derived from the root of the ginseng plant. Most uses have not been fully proven scientifically. Any benefits to teeth and gums have not been substantiated.
Glycerin	Prevents drying out of products.	Derived from palm oil.
Goldenseal	Exerts influence on the mucous surfaces and on the tissues they contact.	Extracted from the root of the goldenseal plant.
Hydrogen peroxide	Disinfects, cleanses, bleaches, and liberates oxygen.	Long-time use is not recommended.
Jojoba	Soothes, may relieve swelling.	Obtained from the jojoba bean. Has no known side effects.
Myrrh	Antiseptic, used to treat halitosis (bad breath).	Obtained from trees and shrubs of the genus *Commiphora*.
Quaternary ammonium compound	Reduces plaque by acting as an antiseptic, solvent, and emulsifying agent. Used in Cepacol and Scope.	Adverse reactions may include a burning sensation in the mouth.
Sage	Astringent.	Extracted from leaves of *salvia officinalis*. An excellent gargle for sore throat. May cause dry mouth.
Sanguinarine	Reduces bacteria's ability to attach to teeth and gums. Also retards the acid-producing ability of bacteria. Used in Viadent toothpaste and mouthwash.	Derived from the bloodroot plant. Chemical name is benzophenathradine. Adverse effects may include a burning sensation in the mouth.
Sodium citrate	Anticoagulant.	A chemical.
Tea tree oil	Said to have antiseptic and antifungal properties. Used in toothpastes found in health-food stores.	Essential oil of the plant *Melaleuca alternifolia*. Research into its benefits has been limited.
Thyme essence	Used in some toothpastes and mouthwashes for its antiseptic action.	Also known as oil of thyme (thymol), an extract of leaves and flowers of *thymus vulgaris*.
Titanium dioxide	A whitening agent used in toothpastes.	TiO_2, derived from titanium, a metallic element.
Witch hazel	Used in mouthwashes for its astringent properties, has a mild anti-inflammatory effect.	Extracted from bark and leaves of the witch hazel shrub.
Zinc chloride	Astringent, used in some mouthwashes.	A mineral.
Zinc oxide	Has mild, soothing astringent properties. Used in some toothpastes.	A mineral.

Diet and Nutrition

We've all heard "you are what you eat." This is, to a large extent, true. Every day, your body renews its structures, building new muscle, bone, skin, and blood. The foods you eat provide the building blocks for these new tissues. In order to accomplish this task, foods must supply energy and nutrients. The six kinds of nutrients are: water, carbohydrates (including fiber), fats, proteins, vitamins, and minerals. These include nutrients that cannot be made by the body but must come from raw materials—food. These essential nutrients include:

- some carbohydrates
- the essential fatty acids (found in fats)
- the essential amino acids (found in proteins)
- fifteen vitamins
- approximately twenty-five minerals
- water

Water is a major constitutent of most of the food we eat. Fats and proteins, which provide the energy and building blocks on which cells depend, are also abundant. The least abundant materials found in foods are vitamins and minerals, but they are no less important. Vitamins are the metabolic regulators and some minerals also serve as building blocks for bones and teeth. If we do not eat enough of the vitamins and minerals we need, our bodies are likely to develop deficiency diseases.

Although poor hygiene plays a major role in the development of gum disease and tooth decay, an extremely important secondary factor is diet and nutrition. In the 1920s and '30s, a dentist by the name of Westen Price studied the relationship between diet and tooth decay. His study compared a modernized community in Switzerland with a more traditional one.

TRADITIONAL VS. MODERN DIET

In the traditional community of Loetschental Valley, life was simple: Cultural and spiritual values were highly appreciated and practiced, and there were no policemen or jails. The people's diet included whole grains harvested locally in the valley, and fresh milk and cheese from their own goats and cows. Dr. Price also found in his tests that the soil was rich in vitamins and minerals.

Dental surveys conducted among the valley's children between the ages of seven and sixteen indicated they had 0.3 cavities per person. In other words, one out of three children had 1 cavity, and two out of three had no cavities! However, Dr. Price's surveys on children in modern communities provided significantly different results. These children, with diets rich in refined flour and sugar, had 20.2 cavities per child. Dr. Price surveyed a third community in which some foods were purchased, but home-grown foods were consumed more frequently. This community had an average of 2.3 cavities per 100 teeth, a little less than 1 cavity per person.

Over the years, Dr. Price conducted the same studies among other peoples such as Native Americans, the Melanesians and Polynesians, tribes in eastern and central Africa, the aborigines of Australia, Alaskan Eskimos, the Maoris of New Zealand, and tribes located in the Amazon basin of Peru. The results always proved the same: There was a definite relationship between the rate of cavities and modern diet.

Dr. Price found that along with the higher incidence

of cavities associated with the modern diet, there was also more crowding of teeth, with the presence of malformed dental arches, malformations of bones in the face and head, personality disturbances, and a greater incidence of other types of diseases. Heredity did not appear to be a contributing factor since Dr. Price found that the problems existed among children who were eating a modern diet, but not among their siblings who had been born before the parents had adopted the new diet.

The new or modern diet consisted of "processed foods," those made with synthetic chemicals for the purpose of improving either taste, appearance, or shelf life. Dr. Price found most of these foods to be lacking in vital nutrients, but high in refined flour and sugar.

Bacteria in the mouth use sugars—sugar, molasses, honey, corn sweeteners, and corn syrups—for energy and to reproduce. When hygiene is poor and the diet is high in sugars, more bacteria is produced, causing an increase in the amount of plaque formed. Bacteria may not respond in the same way to artificial sweeteners such as saccharin or Nutrasweet; however, it remains to be seen what effects these chemicals may have on the rest of the body.

Studies have indicated it is more harmful to eat sugar-containing foods in between meals than it is to eat them with meals. The more the teeth and gums are exposed to the sugars, the more damage is done. In other words, if you eat sweets with your meals, you are exposing your teeth to acid-producing foods two to three times a day. Eating sweets in between meals significantly increases your exposure, since most meals already contain acid-producing ingredients such as meats and breads.

A balanced diet consists of foods that contain the right nutrients for the maintenance of healthy tissues in the body. Soft, sticky foods, which tend to remain on the grooves and in between the teeth, produce more plaque. A diet high in firm fibrous foods such as fruits and vegetables tends to help clean the teeth and tissues. Chewing gums that contain sugar, saccharin, and other chemicals should be avoided.

An honest inventory of your hygiene routine and diet will determine where you need to direct your attention. You should certainly consider the possibility of nutritional deficiencies if you brush and floss every day and still notice bleeding gums, cold sores, and cavities. The lack of certain vitamins, for instance, is revealed by various signs and symptoms in the mouth. To avoid experiencing such symptoms, it is important to learn some basic facts about vitamins. It may be helpful to complete the seven-day survey of your diet on page 16 to determine the nutritional value of your

food. If seven days is too long, try a three- to five-day survey.

VITAMINS

Vitamins are essential to life. Since adequate amounts of vitamins cannot be manufactured within the body, we must get vitamins from foods or supplements. Adequate intake of vitamins, whether from the foods we eat or from added supplements, is essential for healthy teeth and gums. For example, bleeding gums may be the result of a vitamin C deficiency.

The vitamins, in order of their importance for good oral health are: vitamin C, the B vitamins, folic acid, biotin, choline, vitamin D, vitamin A, vitamin E, vitamin K, and coenzyme Q-10. These vitamins are listed below along with information about their effects on the teeth, gums, and supporting structures in the mouth. General recommended dosages are listed here; specific doses for various diseases and disorders are given in Part Two.

BIOTIN

Biotin is a component of a coenzyme that is used in the metabolism of protein and in the synthesis of fat and glycogen. Produced in the gastrointestinal tract by "friendly" bacteria, biotin is thought to decrease muscle pain, depression, and fatigue. However, there are no recognized therapeutic uses for biotin. Deficiency can lead to abnormal heart actions, loss of appetite, nausea, skin rashes, and loss of hair. There are no known toxicity symptoms.

Deficiencies of biotin are rare unless you eat large quantities of raw egg whites, which contain a substance called avidin that prevents absorption of biotin. Biotin is found in brewer's yeast, soybeans, brown rice, butter, lentils, and walnuts.

Precautions and Recommendations

- The Food and Nutrition Board of the National Research Council (NRC) has determined that 100 to 200 micrograms is the estimated safe daily dose for adults. No official recommended daily requirement of biotin has been established for children.

- Excessive amounts of antibiotics and smoking of tobacco may destroy the biotin-producing "friendly" bacteria in the intestines.

CHOLINE

Because it is synthesized in the body, choline is not

DIET SURVEY

It is recommended that adults eat six to eleven servings a day of bread, cereal, rice, and pasta; two to four servings of fruit; three to five servings of vegetables; two to three servings of milk, yogurt, and cheese; and two to three servings of meat, poultry, fish, dry beans, eggs, and nuts. It is recommended that fats, oils, and sweets be used sparingly. Skinless poultry and fish should be consumed more frequently than red meats, which are usually high in fat and calories.

In the survey below, list how often per day you eat each type of food listed.Under the sugar column, list all foods that contain refined sugar.

	Sugar	Milk Products	Meat/Fish/Poultry Dry Beans/Eggs/Nuts	Fruits Vegetables	Bread/Grains
Day 1					
Day 2					
Day 3					
Day 4					
Day 5					
Day 6					
Day 7					

considered an essential vitamin. However, since it is present in meat, eggs, and fish, it is considered a B-complex vitamin. Choline is essential for the use of fats in the body. It prevents fats from being deposited in the liver and helps to move fats into cells. Choline is also a major component of acetylcholine, which is involved in the transmission of nerve signals. Choline deficiency can lead to cirrhosis of the liver, cholesterol deposits in blood vessels, and hardening of the arteries. Organ meats, wheat germ, brewer's yeast, and egg yolks are rich sources of choline.

Precautions and Recommendations

- Although no daily requirements of choline have been established, 400 milligrams per day for adults has been suggested by the Food and Nutrition Board of the NRC. (It is estimated that the average American gets 400 to 900 milligrams a day from dietary sources.) No official recommended daily requirement of choline has been suggested for children.

- The estimated toxic dose of choline is 2000 to 4000 milligrams on a sustained basis. Single doses of up to 10,000 milligrams have not produced any harmful effects.

COENZYME Q-10

A vitamin-like substance that resembles vitamin E, coenzyme Q-10 is a powerful antioxidant. Coenzyme Q-10, which plays a critical role in the effectiveness of the immune system, declines with age and should be supplemented in the diet. Research has shown that use of coenzyme Q-10 benefits allergies, asthma, and respiratory disease. It is also beneficial in combating the effects of aging, candidiasis, diabetes, multiple sclerosis, obesity, and periodontal disease.

Precautions and Recommendations

- Coenzyme Q-10 is generally available in 10 milligram capsules. (Usage over 300 milligrams requires professional guidance.)

- There is no recommended daily allowance for coenzyme Q-10.

- Even in high doses, there are few adverse effects when using coenzyme Q-10. There have, however, been some reports of appetite loss, gastrointestinal upset, diarrhea, and nausea.

FOLIC ACID

Folic acid is important in the development of red blood cells, and works with vitamin B_{12} in the synthesis of RNA (ribonucleic acid) and DNA (deoxyribonucleic acid), cellular carriers of genetic information. Folic acid deficiency results in anemia, with symptoms in the mouth that include swelling of the tongue, cracks in the corners of the mouth, and gum disease. Poor diet, pregnancy, chronic alcoholism, and problems with absorption may cause folic acid deficiency.

Glandular meats such as liver, green leafy vegetables, beans, and seeds contain high levels of folic acid.

Precautions and Recommendations

- According to the Food and Nutrition Board of the NRC, the daily requirement of folic acid for adults is 400 micrograms, with pregnant women requiring an additional 400 micrograms, and lactating women another 100 micrograms. Children require 30 to 300 micrograms.

- Freezing, heating, and canning destroy 50 to 95 percent of the folic acid in foods.

- Anemics and those on anticonvulsive medication or oral contraceptives should consult their physicians before taking folic acid.

VITAMIN A

Vitamin A is a fat-soluble vitamin that occurs in nature in a variety of chemical forms. Vitamin A in the form of retinol is found exclusively in animal tissues, including those of salt-water fishes. Beta-carotene, the precursor of vitamin A, is present in plants and highest in certain fruits, such as apricots and cantaloupes, and in vegetables such as carrots, pumpkins, sweet potatoes, spinach, squash, and broccoli. While retinol is readily absorbed as is by the body, beta-carotene must be broken down in the body before it functions as a vitamin.

Vitamin A is necessary for normal vision and the healthy maintenance of the surface lining (mucous membrane) of the eyes, mouth, and respiratory, intestinal, and genital areas. Deficiency of the vitamin results in impaired vision called night blindness, and thickening of the mucous membranes of the above listed areas. Vitamin A is thought to prevent some cancers, but further research is required to determine how or to what extent it is effective.

Deficiency of vitamin A also leads to dry mouth due

to the vitamin's effects on the salivary glands. Deficiency leads to defective dentin formation since it decreases the activity of new bone cells (osteoblast) and teeth cells, specifically those responsible for the production of dentin (odontoblast). Vitamin A deficiency, therefore, interferes with the growth of bones and teeth. Excessive intake of vitamin A results in a toxic condition characterized by itching skin, gum disease (gingivitis), and irritability. Excess also causes cracked lips and mouth ulcers.

Precautions and Recommendations

- According to the Food and Nutrition Board of the NRC, the recommended daily dose of vitamin A is 5000 IU for adult males, and 4000 IU for women. Pregnant women need an additional 1000 IU, and lactating women require an additional 2000 IU. The recommended daily dose for children is 700 IU.

- Toxicity to this vitamin occurs in adults when doses higher than 50,000 IU are taken daily for an extended period of time.

- Vitamin A in foods or in supplement form is destroyed when exposed to heat, light, and air.

- If you have diabetes, hyperthyroidism, or diseases of the kidney, liver, or pancreas, consult a doctor before taking vitamin A.

- Tobacco, alcohol, and antacids decrease vitamin A absorption.

VITAMIN B₁ (Thiamin)

Thiamin is a water-soluble vitamin that is converted in the liver to an active coenzyme form. Coenzymes are catalysts that enable a chemical reaction to take place, activate the reaction, or speed it up. Thiamin is involved in the release of energy by converting carbohydrates (sugars and starches) into energy in the muscles and nervous system.

A severe deficiency of vitamin B₁ leads to a condition called beriberi. Characteristics of beriberi include muscular weakness, enlargement of the heart, loss of appetite, and constipation. Mild thiamin deficiency symptoms include tiredness, loss of appetite, moodiness, pain, numbness and tingling of the arms and legs, decreased blood pressure, and lowered body temperature. In the mouth, signs of deficiency include burning sensation of the tongue, loss of taste, unusual sensitivity of the inner lining (oral mucosa) of the mouth, and cracks and sores in the corners of the mouth (angular cheilosis).

Foods of both animal and plant origin contain thiamin. Foods richest in thiamin include whole grains such as wheat germ, bran, and oatmeal; and legumes such as peanuts and peas. Meat, fish, fruit, and milk also contain thiamin.

Precautions and Recommendations

- According to the Food and Nutrition Board of the NRC, the average suggested intake of thiamin for an adult is approximately 1.1 to 1.4 milligrams daily. The suggested daily intake for children is 1.2 milligrams, with 1.4 milligrams suggested for pregnant women, and 1.5 milligrams for lactating women.

- If foods are heated above 100°C, the vitamin tends to be destroyed. Prolonged boiling and washing will also destroy the thiamin in foodstuffs. For best results, use steam or minimum water at low temperatures when cooking foods that contain thiamin.

- If you have liver or kidney disease, consult your doctor before taking thiamin.

- Toxic reactions to thiamin are very rare, especially if the vitamin is taken orally rather than by injection. Toxic levels may cause shock or drowsiness.

VITAMIN B₂ (Riboflavin)

Like most B-complex vitamins, riboflavin is involved in the production of energy through the conversion of nutrients in food. Commonly, symptoms of riboflavin deficiency are exhibited in the lip, tongue, eye, and skin areas. The corners of the lips may crack and become painful and ulcerated. The lips may also appear either redder than usual or whitish. Contact with food or drink may cause pain or a burning sensation in the tongue. Small capillaries increase in the cornea, and ulcers may form. The area around the nose, cheeks, and chin may form scales and have a greasy appearance.

This water-soluble vitamin is found in both animal and plant tissues. Meats and dairy products contain the highest amounts of riboflavin. Other sources include bee pollen, almonds, mustard greens, and wheat germ.

Precautions and Recommendations

- The daily minimal requirement for this vitamin set by the Food and Drug Administration (FDA) is 1.2 milligrams. However, the Food and Nutrition Board of the National Research Council (NRC) has set the minimum at 1.2 to 1.7 milligrams, with pregnant women requiring 0.3 milligrams more, and lactating women another 0.5 milligrams. The suggested daily intake for children is 1.4 milligrams.

- Toxic levels of riboflavin are not known. Large doses are passed out of the body via the urine.

- Unlike other water-soluble vitamins, riboflavin is relatively stable to heat, and, therefore, not easily destroyed by cooking.

- People with intestinal diseases have decreased absorption of riboflavin, as do those who use alcohol or tobacco.

- Antidepressants decrease the effects of this vitamin.

VITAMIN B₃ (Niacin)

Niacin (nicotinic acid) and niacinamide (nicotinamide) are water-soluble and chemically different forms of vitamin B₃. However, they have the same basic vitamin activity.

Niacin is involved in the metabolism of carbohydrates and fats by acting as a coenzyme (catalyst) in processes that require energy for normal cell function. Deficiency of this vitamin is mostly seen in areas where the diet consists primarily of corn. Chronic alcoholism, pregnancy, infections, hyperthyroidism, and gastrointestinal disturbances may also cause niacin deficiency. This deficiency produces a disease called pellagra, which is characterized by swollen tongue, inflammation of the mouth, diarrhea, and small, red eruptions on the back of the hands.

As the disease advances, the skin becomes red, thick, and rough. This is followed by scaling. Diarrhea causes the lining of the colon to become inflamed. A burning sensation is experienced in the inner lining of the mouth, and the tongue and lips become red and swollen. Eventually, gum disease characterized by ulcers occurs. Changes in the brain cells and the spinal cord appear and dementia (deterioration of the mental state) follows.

Good sources of niacin are meats, turkey and other poultry; fish such as tuna, salmon, and swordfish; and peanuts.

Precautions and Recommendations

- According to the Food and Nutrition Board of the NRC, daily minimum requirements for adults are 13 to 19 milligrams. Pregnant women require an additional 2 milligrams, and lactating women another 5 milligrams. The suggested daily intake for children is 16 milligrams.

- When a person takes more than 500 milligrams per day of nicotinic acid, a flush described as a burning, stinging sensation is experienced in the hands and face. Other side effects may include upset stomach, vomiting, and diarrhea. Liver damage may result with prolonged use.

- Consult your doctor before taking niacin if you have diabetes, or gall bladder or liver disease.

VITAMIN B₅ (Pantothenic Acid)

This water-soluble vitamin is converted in the body to a catalyst called coenzyme A. The breakdown of fatty acids, metabolism of carbohydrates, conversion of glycogen to glucose, and steroid hormones require coenzyme A.

Deficiencies of pantothenic acid are extremely rare. However, experimentally induced deficiencies have produced fatigue, headache, nausea, abdominal pain, and cramping of leg muscles. Pantothenic acid is considered nontoxic. Doses as high as 10,000 milligrams daily have revealed no side effects.

Since pantothenic acid is available in all living material, most diets contain adequate amounts. Some of the best sources are corn, egg yolk, liver, lentils, and nuts.

Precautions and Recommendations

- Although no daily requirements have been established in humans, the Food and Nutrition Board of the NRC has suggested that adults get 5 to 10 milligrams of pantothenic acid each day.

- Tobacco use decreases the absorption of vitamin B₅.

VITAMIN B₆ (Pyridoxine)

Pyridoxine is usually associated with vitamin B₆; however, this vitamin actually consists of three substances: pyridoxine, pyridoxal phosphate, and pyridoxamine. Pyridoxal phosphate is manufactured in our bodies from pyridoxine and is utilized in the formation of amino acids, which are the building blocks for proteins. Pyridoxal phosphate is also needed for proper central nervous system function and is involved in the manufacture of hemoglobin, which is responsible for the transfer of oxygen from the lungs to the cells in the body.

While severe deficiencies of pyridoxine are rare, mild cases have been produced with a diet poor in vitamin B complex. The symptoms associated with a deficiency of the B complex resemble those associated with deficiencies of riboflavin, niacin, and thiamin. These include cracks at the corners of the mouth, and itching and scaling around the nose and chin area.

Most foods of plant and animal origin contain this vitamin. Most vegetables are rich sources of pyridoxine, while pyridoxal phosphate and pyridoxamine are found in animal products. Cereal grains, milk, meat, and avocados are excellent sources of vitamin B6.

Precautions and Recommendations

- The Food and Nutrition Board of the NRC has set the daily requirement of vitamin B6 for adults at 1.8 to 2.2 milligrams, with an additional 0.6 milligrams required for pregnant women, and an additional 0.5 milligrams required for lactating women. The suggested daily recommendation for children is 1.6 milligrams.

- Doses up to 100 milligrams daily are nontoxic. Prolonged (more than one month) administration of 200 milligrams or more daily may cause symptoms similar to deficiency symptoms caused by abruptly ceasing vitamin supplements.

- Vitamin B6 cancels the therapeutic effects of levodopa, which is used for the treatment of Parkinson's disease.

- Deficiencies have been produced in women taking estrogenic steroids.

- *The Journal of the Canadian Psychiatric Association* published a report in 1973 by J.V. Ananth, who indicated that vitamin B6 enhances the therapeutic effectiveness of nicotinic acid in the treatment of schizophrenia.

VITAMIN B12 (Cyanocobalamine)

Vitamin B12 is not found in plants, but in bacteria that are eaten by animal species and available for human consumption. Vitamin B12 is not absorbed without the presence of a protein-binding factor called intrinsic factor, which is secreted by the lining of the stomach. When this factor is missing, vitamin B12 is not absorbed, and pernicious anemia (insufficient red blood cells caused by dietary deficiencies) or Addison's disease (life-threatening disease caused by failure of the adrenal glands) results. Another cause of vitamin B12 deficiency is inadequate dietary intake, which is a consideration for vegetarians. Signs of deficiency in the mouth include soreness and burning of the tongue, and painful, bright red sores that occur on the inner lining of the cheeks and the undersurface of the tongue. Vitamin B12 is generally considered nontoxic.

Vitamin B12 supplements are available in multivitamins and in B-complex preparations. Physicians may also administer B12 by injection.

Precautions and Recommendations

- According to the Food and Nutrition Board of the NRC, the recommended daily dose of vitamin B12 for adults is 3 micrograms, with pregnant and lactating women requiring an additional 1 microgram. The suggested daily recommendation for children is 3 micrograms.

- If you have gout, consult your doctor before taking this vitamin.

- If large doses of vitamin C are taken along with B12, side effects such as nosebleeds, bleeding from the ear, or dry mouth may result.

VITAMIN C (Ascorbic Acid)

Water-soluble vitamin C aids in the formation of collagen, which is a constituent of all connective tissue. Since connective tissue is an important component of the gums, vitamin C is necessary for the maintenance of healthy gums and for proper healing after tooth extraction or gum surgery. Because of its effects on the bone matrix, vitamin C deficiency can lead to mild or severe tooth loosening and tooth loss.

Deficiency symptoms of vitamin C are related to the inability of the connective tissue to produce collagen, bone matrix, dentin, cartilage, and blood vessel walls (vascular endothelium.) These symptoms include poor healing; inadequate walling of infection, so that infections may spread more easily; weakened blood vessel walls, which cause excess bleeding in the skin, gums, lungs, muscles, and joints, and a tendency to bruise easily; and inadequately formed bone matrix, which causes weak bones and resorption of the bone supporting the teeth, resulting in loosening and loss of teeth. Vitamin C deficiency also causes extremely dry mouth, which can contribute to cavities and gum disease.

Fresh fruits and vegetables—including citrus fruits, green vegetables, tomatoes, and berries—are rich sources of vitamin C.

Precautions and Recommendations

- According to the Food and Nutrition Board of the NRC, adult daily requirements of Vitamin C are 60 milligrams, with pregnant and lactating women requiring 20 to 40 milligrams more. Children are recommended to take 45 to 50 milligrams daily.

- Doses of 1 gram or more of vitamin C can produce diarrhea, flushed face, nausea, and vomiting.

- To conserve the vitamin C found in foods, eat them raw or minimally cooked. (Cooking in copper pots and prolonged cooking in water destroys vitamin C.) Avoid soaking vegetables for long periods.

- Avoid chewing vitamin C tablets, which may promote decay due to acid residue left on teeth.

VITAMIN D

Vitamin D is produced by the interaction of the sun's ultraviolet rays with oils of the skin. By increasing the blood level of minerals, particularly calcium and phosphorus, vitamin D permits bone formation and maintenance. Vitamin D deficiency in children causes "rickets," which is characterized by overgrowth of cartilage, resulting in weak, soft bone that easily bends and fractures. Bone pain and muscle weakness may also be present. Children with rickets show severe disturbances in the teeth and jaws; for example, teeth erupting late, crooked teeth, and underdeveloped lower jaw. In adults, rickets is known as osteomalacia. The condition occurs among women with low calcium intake and little exposure to sun, who have repeatedly breastfed.

Food products with vitamin D include milk and fish-liver oils. Vitamin D supplements are available as cholecalciferol and ergocalciferol. Vitamin D is highly toxic. Toxicity symptoms can occur with ingestion of just four to five times the recommended daily allowance.

Precautions and Recommendations

- According to the Food and Nutrition Board of the NRC, the recommended daily allowance of vitamin D for infants up to the age of six months is 7.5 micrograms (300 IU); for those over the age of six months, 10 micrograms (400 IU) is recommended. For adults up to age twenty-five, the daily recommendation is 10 micrograms, with those over age twenty-five requiring only 5 micrograms (200 IU). An additional 5 micrograms is recommended for pregnant and lactating women.

- Vitamin D toxicity is associated with daily intakes of 2000 IU. Symptoms include weakness, fatigue, headache, nausea, vomiting, and diarrhea. Toxic levels are related to hypercalcemia, which may result in calcification of blood vessels, heart, lungs, and kidneys. Continued overdose can lead to calcium deposits in soft tissues such as the kidneys and heart. In the latter case, death can result.

VITAMIN E

Three substances—alpha, beta, and gamma tocopherol—were initially isolated from wheat germ, and collectively are referred to as vitamin E. Alpha tocopherol is considered the most important of the three substances since it is involved in more biological activities than the other two.

Although numerous claims are made about the role of vitamin E, many of them are based on incomplete evidence. The vitamin does appear to have an active role as an antioxidant. Antioxidants have the ability to protect delicate structures in the cells from attack by "free radicals." These free radicals are harmful and often cause injury to the cellular structures, literally burning them. Ozone, nitrogen dioxide, and high concentrations of oxygen contain these free radicals.

Deficiency of vitamin E is often seen in individuals who have problems with absorption such as in Crohn's disease, and in children with cystic fibrosis. Vitamin E deficiencies may also be seen in people who for years have eliminated fats from their diets, and in individuals who eat primarily highly processed foods. It has been suggested that when a vitamin E deficiency exists, degenerative changes occur in the skeletal muscle cells, and leg cramps and fibrocystic breast disease may occur. Excellent sources of vitamin E include soybean, corn, and cottonseed oils; green vegetables; and wheat germ.

Vitamin E is far less toxic than the other fat-soluble vitamins. A daily intake in the range of 200 to 800 IU per day is generally considered safe.

Precautions and Recommendations

- The recommended daily allowance for vitamin E is expressed in alpha tocopherol equivalents. According to the Food and Nutrition Board of the NRC, the adult daily intake of vitamin E should fall between 7 and 13 IU alpha tocopherol equivalents. The daily intake for children should fall between 3 and 7 IU.

- Nausea and diarrhea have been reported at dosage levels in excess of 1000 IU.

- Natural tocopherols are relatively unstable and lose significant activity during storage and cooking.

- Vitamin E appears to increase the vitamin K requirement, and megadoses of vitamin E administered together with the anticoagulant drug warfarin may result in heavy bleeding.

- Vitamin E may help strengthen weak muscles in temporomandibular joint dysfunction (TMJ).

VITAMIN K

Vitamin K, a fat-soluble vitamin, is involved in the synthesis of at least two proteins necessary for blood clotting. Severe deficiency of vitamin K may result in heavy bleeding even from minor trauma. A vitamin K deficiency is usually caused by inadequate intake and poor absorption of the vitamin.

There are two forms of Vitamin K. Vitamin K_1 (phylloquinone) occurs in green vegetables such as alfalfa, cabbage, and spinach, and in egg yolks, soybean oil, and liver. Vitamin K_2 (menaquinone) is synthesized by intestinal microorganisms such as bacteria. It is believed that people obtain about half of their daily needs from the vitamin K synthesized by "friendly" bacteria.

The best sources of vitamin K are turnip greens, broccoli, Brussels sprouts, spinach, and lettuce. Liver, bacon, cheese, butter, coffee, and green tea have moderate amounts of this vitamin. The natural vitamins K_1 and K_2 are nontoxic even in massive doses. The synthetic form, called menadione, is relatively nontoxic but can be toxic, especially to newborns and pregnant women.

Precautions and Recommendations

- The Food and Nutrition Board of the NRC has set the recommended daily allowance of vitamin K at 100 micrograms for adults. The range for children is 5 to 30 micrograms.

- At birth, babies usually receive a small dose of vitamin K, since their intestines are sterile and lack the necessary amounts normally provided by the intestinal bacteria.

- Use of aspirin, mineral oil, antibiotics, and sulfa drugs, and exposure to x-rays or air pollutants can lead to a deficiency of vitamin K.

MINERALS

Minerals are substances that are not of animal or plant origin. They are found in nature and are essential constituents of all cells. Minerals form the greater portion of the hard parts of the body: bone, teeth, and nails. They serve many functions, including regulating permeability of cell membranes and capillaries, regulating reaction and activity of muscular and nervous tissue, and ensuring acid-base balance. Minerals are important components of glandular secretions, and are essential in water metabolism and in the regulation of blood volume.

Minerals are excreted daily from the body. Because they cannot be synthesized by organisms, they must be replaced through food intake. Maintenance of the normal concentration of minerals is essential to plant life as well as animal and even bacterial life.

Minerals can be divided into two types or classes—major and trace. Major minerals, or macrominerals, are required in the diet at levels in excess of 100 milligrams per day and include, in order of their importance to dental health, calcium, phosphorus, magnesium, sodium, potassium, chloride, and sulfur. Trace minerals, or microminerals, are required in the diet at levels much less than 100 milligrams per day. In order of their importance to dental health, the trace minerals include iron, zinc, iodine, selenium, chromium, manganese, copper, cobalt, and fluoride. The major and trace minerals are discussed below.

CALCIUM

Approximately 99 percent of the calcium—the structural component of bone, enamel, and cementum—in an adult's body is found in bones and teeth. Calcium is also involved in normal clotting of blood, muscle contraction, heart and nerve function, and hormone release. Adequate intake of calcium is obviously essential to well-being. If daily intake falls below 500 milligrams, calcium is absorbed from bone to be used for these functions. A calcium deficiency can cause increased muscle and nerve irritability, tremors, convulsions, rickets, and osteomalacia (softening of the bones). Excess amounts of calcium (hypercalcemia) are either stored in bone or excreted in urine. Prolonged excess can cause confusion, irregular heartbeat, bone cysts, and impaired kidney function.

Calcium metabolism is influenced by calcitonin (a parathyroid hormone) and vitamin D. Calcitonin is the most important regulator of calcium levels. When high levels of this hormone are produced, as with an overactive parathyroid gland, calcium is not absorbed properly, and weakness and bone fractures can result. Vitamin D controls the absorption of calcium from the small intestine and plays a role in calcium resorption in the kidneys. Due to vitamin D deficiency and its effect on calcium, eruption of teeth may be delayed and gum disease may be present. Once teeth have erupted, the amount of calcium in them remains unchanged. The jaw, however, is one of the first things affected when there is a calcium deficiency, as the mineral is drawn out of the jawbone. Although some loss of bone density in the jaw is a normal consequence of the aging process, improper habits are also contributing factors.

Osteoporosis, a decrease in bone mass that causes

skeletal weakness and has been linked to calcium deficiency, is a disorder that is frequently associated with postmenopausal women. When osteoporosis is present, there is an increased risk of jaw fracture during pulling of teeth. Healing after tooth extraction may also be delayed. Also, due to the thinning of bone, it may be difficult to make dentures fit properly.

Rich sources of calcium include seaweed, sesame seeds, molasses, Swiss cheese, and other dairy products. Calcium supplements are known as calcium salts and are available in the following combinations: calcium gluconate, calcium lactate, calcium carbonate, calcium glubionate, and dibasic calcium phosphate dihydrate. The amount of pure calcium in each form of these combinations varies. Calcium carbonate contains 40 percent pure calcium, while calcium gluconate contains 9 percent; calcium lactate contains 13 percent; calcium glubionate, 6.5 percent; and dibasic calcium phosphate dihydrate, 23 percent pure calcium. These figures mean that 1000 milligrams of calcium carbonate contain 400 milligrams of calcium, while 1000 milligrams of calcium glubionate contain only 6.5 percent pure calcium.

Precautions and Recommendations

- It is recommended by the Food and Nutrition Board of the NRC, that adults obtain 800 to 1200 milligrams of calcium daily, with children receiving 800 milligrams, and pregnant and lactating women obtaining 1600 milligrams.

- Calcium supplements are often used to treat hypocalcemia and acid stomach. The use of dolomite—a magnesium and calcium carbonate complex mined from the ground—is not recommended. The FDA has found lead contamination in this form.

- Studies have indicated that when daily calcium intake of older women was increased to 800 milligrams per day over a three-year period, their bones became more dense and, therefore, stronger.

- Calcium supplements should be avoided if digitalis drugs are being taken to prevent heart failure.

- Calcium decreases the absorption of the antibiotic tetracycline.

- If large doses of calcium are taken for long periods of time, kidney stones may form.

CHLORIDE

Chloride is found in the fluid outside cells in combination with sodium. Inside cells, chloride is usually found in association with potassium. This means that chloride is necessary for the maintenance of fluid balances in the body. It is also a constituent of hydrochloric acid and is, therefore, necessary for proper digestion.

We get almost all of our chloride from the sodium chloride in foods and beverages. Deficiency can be caused by excessive sweating, chronic diarrhea, or vomiting. Chloride deficiency can cause growth failure in children, muscle cramps, mental apathy, and loss of appetite. Excess chloride is excreted by the kidneys and skin. Consistent excesses of chloride have been linked to high blood pressure in some people. Chloride toxicity is rare but can cause vomiting.

Precautions and Recommendations

- No recommended allowance has been established for chloride; but, a safe and adequate daily level is estimated to be from 1700 to 5100 milligrams.

CHROMIUM

Chromium is believed necessary to maintain normal glucose metabolism, which generates energy.

The active form of chromium is known as "glucose tolerance factor" (GTF), and is found in high concentrations in brewer's yeast. Oysters, eggs, calves liver, American cheese, and wheat germ are other good sources of chromium.

Chromium has no known deficiency conditions or toxic levels. It is thought that chromium deficiency may impair glucose tolerance in malnourished children and some diabetics.

Precautions and Recommendations

- The Food and Nutrition Board of the NRC recommends .2 milligrams chromium per day for adults, and .08 milligrams for children.

- Consumption of a varied and balanced diet helps to assure adequate and safe chromium intake.

COBALT

Cobalt is a functional component of vitamin B_{12}, which is necessary for the formation of red blood cells. Green leafy vegetables are the richest source of cobalt. Cobalt deficiency may cause anemia in children. Severe cobalt deficiency has been linked with lack of appetite and emaciation. Toxic levels of cobalt may cause cardiomyopathy (a disease that affects the heart muscles), elevated hemoglobin, coma, and even death.

Precautions and Recommendations

- No minimum daily requirements for cobalt have been established.

- Ingestion of inorganic cobalt may be important to strict vegetarians, whose ability to maintain B12 levels is limited.

COPPER

Copper works with iron in the formation of hemoglobin. It is also a constituent of collagen (connective tissue) and of many enzymes. Although dietary copper deficiency is not known to occur in adults, it has been seen in malnourished children in Peru. Liver, seafood, nuts, and seeds are the richest sources of dietary copper. Food and supplemental intake of copper greater than 10 milligrams per day may result in toxicity, causing nausea, vomiting, and stomach pains.

Precautions and Recommendations

- The Food and Nutrition Board of the NRC does not list recommended daily allowances for copper, but estimates adequate amounts to be 1.5 to 3 milligrams per day for adults, and 1 to 2 milligrams for children.

- Some studies have indicated a positive relationship between the zinc-copper ratio in the diet and the incidence of cardiovascular disease.

FLUORIDE

Although fluoride is not called an essential element, it is considered beneficial because of its valuable effects on dental health. Most of the body's fluoride is found in the bones and teeth, and fluoride has been recognized as a means to prevent dental cavities if taken at the pre-eruptive stage of the teeth. Further protection is provided by topical application of fluoride during the developmental stage. Teeth that contain fluoride have been shown to be more cavity resistant, and bones containing fluoride are less prone to resorption.

The fluoride content of foods varies, depending on the amount of fluoride in the water where the foods are grown. The richest dietary sources of fluoride are tea and certain fish, such as anchovies and sardines, that are eaten along with their bones. Excess accumulation of fluoride (fluorosis) causes chalky-white irregularly distributed patches on tooth enamel. Severe fluorosis will weaken the enamel and cause surface pitting. Prolonged excessive levels of fluoride can cause osteosclerosis in adults, as well as bony tumors on the spine. Fluoride deficiency may predispose people to cavities and osteoporosis.

Precautions and Recommendations

- The Food and Nutrition Board of the NRC has recommended a daily intake of 1.5 to 4 milligrams of fluoride for adults. To prevent mottling of teeth, children and adolescents from the age of four should have no more than 2.5 milligrams per day. During the first year of life, children should have 0.1 to 1 milligram; during the second year of life, 0.5 to 1.5 milligrams. Water content must be maintained at levels no less than 1 milligram per liter to meet these requirements.

- The Food and Nutrition Board recommends fluoridation of public water supplies when natural levels are less than 0.7 milligrams per liter.

- Fluoride's effect on preventing cavities is greatest during the first eight years of a person's life.

- Excess amounts of fluoride in the diet (20 to 80 milligrams) can adversely affect bones, kidney function, and possibly muscle and nerve function.

- Some suggest that cooking in Teflon-treated pots and pans can increase the fluoride content of food because Teflon contains fluoride. On the other hand, cooking on aluminum surfaces may reduce the amount of fluoride in foods.

IODINE

Iodine is best known for its role in the development and functioning of the thyroid gland, which is the regulator of body metabolism. Iodine is present in food and water as iodide, which is quickly absorbed and transported to the thyroid. There it is synthesized into thyroid hormones.

Excess amounts of iodine may cause allergic reactions, a metallic taste, burning in the mouth and throat, soreness of teeth and gums, increased salivation, and inflammation of the pharynx, larynx, and tonsils. Iodine deficiency in the diet may lead to simple goiter, which is characterized by thyroid enlargement. During prenatal development, iron deficiency may cause cretinism. This congenital condition is characterized in childhood by dwarfed stature, mental retardation, dystrophy of the bones, and a low basal metabolism.

The richest sources of iodine are vegetables that grow near the seacoast, seafoods (especially fish-liver oil), and iodized salt.

Precautions and Recommendations

- According to the NRC's Food and Nutrition Board, the recommended daily requirement of iodine for adults is .15 milligrams, and is increased to .17 milligrams during pregnancy and .2 milligrams during lactation. The daily recommendation for children is .07 milligrams.

- People who live in inland areas where dietary and environmental levels of iodine are low should use iodized salt.

- Iodine is frequently used as an antiseptic for cuts and wounds.

IRON

In the adult body, the highest concentration of iron (60 to 70 percent) is found in hemoglobin (the red part of blood cells). The iron in the body helps hemoglobin transport oxygen and works with enzymes to utilize oxygen for metabolism. Small but essential amounts of iron are also located in muscle in the form of myoglobin.

Because iron is absorbed with difficulty, iron deficiency is one of the most common deficiencies known to human beings. It is most prevalent in women who are menstruating or pregnant. In the latter case, significant amounts of iron are required for building the blood volume of the infant. Symptoms of iron deficiency anemia include weakness, pallor, and reduced resistance to infection. The tongue becomes smooth, giving it a bald appearance, due to alterations to the taste buds and destruction of the papillae (projections) surrounding them. These alterations cause sensitivity to a variety of tastes. Iron overload can cause cirrhosis, diabetes mellitus, and change in skin pigmentation.

Seaweed is the richest source of iron, followed by meat such as liver, pumpkin and sesame seeds, wheat germ, dried pears and other fruits, nuts, and seafood.

Precautions and Recommendations

- The Food and Nutrition Board of the NRC lists the recommended daily allowance for iron as 6 to 10 milligrams for children; 10 to 12 milligrams for adult males; 15 milligrams for adult females; and 10 milligrams for postmenopausal women.

- Antacids and certain antibiotics, such as tetracycline, decrease the amount of iron absorbed into the blood.

MAGNESIUM

Magnesium is included as one of the three most important elements in bone and teeth, calcium and phosphorus being the other two. In the adult body, 60 percent of the magnesium is found in bone, and 20 percent in muscle. The remainder is involved in other essential functions. Magnesium plays an important role in muscle contraction and relaxation, transmission of nerve impulses, and the release and transfer of energy. Magnesium salts are essential in nutrition, being required for the activity of many enzymes.

Magnesium is a naturally occurring element on Earth. It is found in wells and sea water. Rich sources include molasses, nuts, fish, and whole grains. Magnesium is available as magnesium sulfate, magnesium gluconate, and magnesium-protein complex.

The proper level of magnesium is remarkably constant in healthy people. Deficiencies occur in certain disease states, such as long-term diarrhea, renal dysfunction, and alcoholism. Magnesium toxicity can cause low blood pressure, respiratory failure, and cardiac disturbance.

Precautions and Recommendations

- According to the Food and Nutrition Board of the NRC, the daily dietary allowance of magnesium for adults is 300 to 400 milligrams; pregnant women require 450 milligrams; and children, 50 to 350 milligrams.

- Magnesium is often used as a laxative. Overuse may cause magnesium toxicity.

- Bone meal—a powder of animal bones used to supplement calcium, magnesium, and phosophorus—should be taken with caution because the toxic metals deposited in bone may appear in this supplement.

- Excessive muscle relaxation may result if magnesium is taken during treatment with muscle-relaxing drugs.

- The effectiveness of anticoagulant drugs and certain tranquilizers such as thorazine may be decreased by the use of magnesium supplements.

MANGANESE

Manganese—a component of enzymes used for synthesis and breakdown of carbohydrates, fats, and amino acids—is essential for normal bone structure. Deficiency of manganese may be related to abnormal formation of bone and cartilage, and growth retardation. Neurologic disturbances have been related to toxic levels of manganese in those who work with the ore. Rich sources of manganese include unrefined cereals, green leafy vegetables, and tea.

Precautions and Recommendations

- The daily requirements of manganese are not known, but 2.5 to 5 micrograms per day have been found to be adequate.

- Because manganese deficiency has been observed only in institutionalized populations, the National Research Council has stated that current dietary intakes appear to satisfy the need for manganese.

PHOSPHORUS

Like calcium, phosphorus is an important element in bone, enamel, and cementum. Approximately 80 to 85 percent of the phosphorus in an adult's body is contained in bones and teeth, chiefly in combination with calcium. Phosphorus is also found in muscle (10 percent) and in nerve tissue (1 percent). Vitamin D is important in the metabolism and absorption of phosphorus, which takes place in the intestines. Dietary phosphorus that is not absorbed by the cells is eliminated in urine and feces. Phosphorus is also involved in the body's utilization of fats, proteins, and carbohydrates (sugar). Blood fats combine with phosphorus to form phospholipids, which are a fundamental part of all cells. Phosphorus also combines with amino acids to aid in the production of energy.

An excess of phosphorus in the blood is called hyperphosphatemia. This condition is always present in hypoparathyroidism. When the parathyroid glands are underactive, there is a deficiency of parathyroid hormone, the hormone that helps maintain the calcium and phosphorus levels of the blood. Insufficient levels of these minerals can result in a decrease in bone density.

Long-term poisoning with phosphorus compounds causes a persistent and progressive osteomyelitis (inflammation of bone) of the upper (maxilla) and lower (mandible) jaws. Symptoms of this disorder include pain and pressure over the affected part of the jaw, fever, and sweats.

Phosphorus is a nonmetallic element found in almost all foods. Dairy products, meats, and fish are rich sources, as are nuts, legumes, and grains. However, the phosphorus in nuts, legumes, and grains is not well absorbed because it is tied to insoluble material.

Precautions and Recommendations

- For adults, the recommended daily intake of phosphorus is the same as the recommendation for calcium: 800 to 1200 milligrams. For children, the daily recommendation is 240 to 800 milligrams.

- Alcoholics are prone to phosphorus deficiency due to inadequate dietary intake, vomiting, and diarrhea.

- Excessive use of antacids containing aluminum hydroxide also inhibits phosphate absorption from the intestines, and may be a cause of phosphorus deficiency if the diet is not well balanced.

- Soft drinks contain phosphorus, and high intake of sodas may cause an imbalance of this macromineral.

POTASSIUM

Along with sodium and chloride, potassium aids in regulation of the balance of water inside and outside cells. Potassium is important in the transmission of nerve impulses, the control of skeletal muscle contractility, and the maintenance of normal blood pressure. Severe potassium deficiency can cause paralysis and cardiac disturbances. Potassium toxicity can cause the same conditions. The best sources of potassium are fruits, vegetables, and fresh meats.

Precautions and Recommendations

- No recommended daily allowance has been established for potassium; however, a safe and adequate level is estimated to be from 1875 to 5100 milligrams daily.

- Certain diuretics and adrenal cortical hormones may cause potassium depletion. Consult your physician about potassium intake if you have kidney disease.

SELENIUM

Selenium, which is found in all tissues, works in conjunction with vitamin E to protect bodily compounds that might be destroyed by the effects of oxidation. Selenium deficiency in humans is almost unknown; however, Keshan's disease, a fatal heart disease seen in children living in China, may be due to selenium deficiency. Toxic levels of selenium may cause hair and nail loss, as well as high rates of cavities (caries) in teeth if the selenium was taken during tooth development.

Good sources of selenium include kidney, liver, and seafood. Grains are also a good source, but the selenium content is variable depending on the content of the soil in which the grain is grown.

Precautions and Recommendations

- Selenium requirements have not been established; but an adequate level is estimated to be 50 to 200 micrograms for adults.

- The refining of foods and lengthy cooking times decrease selenium in foods.

- Toxicity can be caused by long-term use of selenium supplements.

SODIUM

Sodium salts are found in the fluids of the body—serum (the clear fluid obtained when whole blood is separated into solid and liquid), blood, and lymph. Sodium helps to maintain the normal fluid balance in cells and the acid-base balance in the body. It is also necessary for transmission of nerve impulses.

High levels of sodium in the diet play a role in high blood pressure (hypertension) and contribute to edema (excessive amount of fluid in body tissues). Foods and beverages that contain sodium chloride (table salt) are a primary source of sodium.

Precautions and Recommendations

- Daily requirements have not been set, but the Food and Nutrition Board of the NRC estimates 500 milligrams of sodium to be the minimum adult daily intake, with a maximum intake of 2400 milligrams.

- Excessive sweating will cause loss of sodium, which may result in an improper amount of water inside and outside cells.

- Sodium bicarbonate (baking soda) is ingested to treat acidosis (abnormal increase of acids). It is also used externally as an alkaline wash. Many toothpastes and mouthwashes contain sodium bicarbonate. Continuous use of such products may cause the pH of the mouth to be more alkaline than acid.

SULFUR

Sulfur is part of the protein in every cell of the body and occurs in most food proteins. Keratin—the protein in hair and nails—is rich in sulfur. Sulfur also occurs in the vitamins biotin and thiamin, and in the hormone insulin. Deficiencies are not known. Toxicity might occur if protein amino acids are ingested in excess.

Foods containing sulfur include Brussels sprouts, dried beans, cabbage, eggs, fish, garlic, and onions. Sulfur may also be obtained from the amino acid supplements L-methionine, L-cysteine, L-lysine, and L-cystine.

Precautions and Recommendations

- No recommended allowance has been established for sulfur.

- Sulfur is not utilized as the free mineral, but through its incorporation into methionine.

ZINC

In the human body, zinc is found in all human tissues and fluids, but is highly concentrated in teeth, bones, hair, skin, liver, muscle, and testes. Zinc is involved in the making of genetic material and proteins. It is part of the hormone insulin and of many enzymes. Zinc influences immune reactions, taste perception, wound healing, and the making of sperm.

Zinc deficiency can cause growth failure in children, retardation of sexual maturation, and poor wound healing. Toxicity symptoms include fever, nausea, vomiting, diarrhea, muscle incoordination, and dizziness. Toxicity can lead to anemia, accelerated atherosclerosis, and kidney failure. Rich sources of zinc include red meats, shellfish, turkey, and wheat germ.

Precautions and Recommendations

- According to the Food and Nutrition Board of the NRC, the recommended daily allowance for zinc is 15 milligrams for adults, which is increased to 20 milligrams during pregnancy and 25 milligrams during breastfeeding. Children's requirements are 3 milligrams daily.

- Zinc levels tend to fall during times of stress or when trauma, infectious diseases, or large doses of steroid drugs are present.

- Increased loss and impaired utilization of zinc are caused by even moderate amounts of alcohol.

- Individuals with oral cancer are often supplemented with up to 100 milligrams of zinc daily to help improve taste perception.

MINOR TRACE MINERALS

Molybdenum, cadmium, nickel, silicon, vanadium, and tin have been identified as trace minerals. Since no known relationship exists between these trace minerals and dental care, they will not be discussed. However, nickel is a component of many metals used in dentistry; and some studies suggest a possible allergic response to this mineral in some individuals.

Homeopathy

When illness affects our bodies, there are other forms of treatment available besides the medications prescribed by physicians. Although prescription drugs are very important in many instances, they can have adverse—sometimes even deadly—side effects. A better understanding of treatment options will enable us to work with our health-care providers to choose the treatment most likely to bring about health in a given situation.

Homeopathy is a treatment option that was practiced widely in the United States until the early twentieth century, when medicinal (pharmaceutical) drugs became popular. Homeopathy is still very much accepted and used in Europe, especially in Germany, Switzerland, and England.

Homeopathy seeks cures that correspond with the natural laws of healing. The living human being is affected by internal as well as external elements, which together result in a dynamic balance or imbalance of the person's mind, body, and spirit. These three parts of the whole are closely interrelated, and whatever happens to one part may ultimately affect one or both of the other parts. The natural laws of healing recognize this principle and the ability of the body to heal itself with the aid of materials and methods that are nontoxic and have no side effects.

The term homeopathy comes from the Greek roots *homoios*, meaning similar, and *pathos*, meaning suffering or sickness. The basic law of homeopathy is "the law of similars." The law states that a substance can cure a disease if it produces in a healthy person symptoms similar to and much milder than those of the disease.

Samuel Christian Friedrich Hahnemann was the German physician who formulated the theory of homeopathy in the 1800s. However, Hahnemann was not the first to discover the concept. In 400 B.C., Hippocrates wrote that through the like, disease is produced, and through application of the like, disease is cured. Besides Hippocrates, Paracelsus, a sixteenth century German physician, also described the law of similars in his writings. However, it was Hahnemann who developed the therapeutic agents prescribed in homeopathy that have been published in the *Materia Medica*. First published in 1927, the *Materia Medica*, by William Boericke, M.D., is the most complete encyclopedia of homeopathic therapeutic agents developed by Hahnemann, and is widely used by homeopathic physicians as a source book.

Today, a homeopathic physician, by observing symptoms of a disease, prescribes the appropriate substance, which under scientifically controlled conditions has produced the same disease symptoms in a healthy person. The traditional form of treating with homeopathic substances was prescribing one therapeutic agent at a time, until the original symptoms had decreased. Some modern practitioners recommend using multiple agents simultaneously. Homeopathic treatments have been found to have no side effects; however, if an inappropriate therapy is given, no change will occur in the symptoms or disease.

Homeopathic therapies are prepared by potentization. Each agent is prepared by successive dilutions of the ingredients (plant or animal origin), alternating with succussion (vigorous shaking), which is continued until the resulting medicine contains no molecules of the original substance. Potencies for homeopathic agents are designated by a number that is followed by an x. The x represents 10, and signifies that the mother tincture has been diluted to one part in 10. The number preceding the x indicates the number of times the remedy has been diluted. The more diluted a remedy is, the more potent it is said to be. Thus, a 6x potency remedy, which has been diluted 6 times, is considered more potent than a 3x remedy, which has been diluted only 3 times.

Sometimes, upon successful treatment of symptoms of the disease, another set of symptoms appears. This is not unusual during homeopathic treatment. Symptoms are the body's methods of protection; they warn that an imbalance exists. Some of the symptoms are really the body's means of restoring harmony. For example, bad breath is a sign that either decay, gum disease, or digestive problems are present. If you choose the appropriate therapy for the bad breath and resolve the problem, you may begin to have symptoms relating to either the digestive system or the teeth, depending on the cause of the bad breath. Sensitive teeth may indicate excessive wear of the enamel due to grinding or clenching of the teeth. This habit may be the result of stress or other factors that should be addressed. If the sensitivity is treated, you may begin to experience other symptoms related to the original cause of the problem. These symptoms may be emotional or physical. Once one set of obvious symptoms related to a disease is treated, a deeper level of symptoms appears, until all underlying causes are addressed. Ultimately, the immune system, which is the body's defense mechanism, must be made strong enough to handle any harmful external attack, whether emotional or physical.

HOMEOPATHIC PREPARATIONS

Homeopathic agents used in treatment and listed in the following table may be purchased from health-food stores. Some homeopathic agents are sold by the name of the illness—"Flu," "PMS," "Asthma," "Cough," "Allergies," etc. These homeopathics have more than one therapeutic agent in them. Other preparations offer single therapies. Due to the manner in which homeopathics work, the single therapy may be the choice, initially. Once you understand how you respond to a particular substance, you can read the labels of the compounded therapies, and choose one of them.

You should have a copy of the *Materia Medica* on hand (available at some health-food stores). Look up the various therapies listed, and determine which may

be best for you, by considering the symptoms that the particular substance treats. It is important to note that mint and coffee may decrease the effectiveness of homeopathic substances.

Consult with your physician before giving homeopathics to children, or before taking them during pregnancy or when breastfeeding. Of course, there are many excellent homeopathic physicians available. Some health-food stores have lists of these physicians, some of whom may also be listed in your *Yellow Pages* under "Physicians." Some osteopathic physicians have also been trained in homeopathic medicine by their medical schools. However, many of these schools stopped teaching homeopathy in the 1950s. Physicians and osteopathic physicians trained in homeopathics are the health-care providers of choice, since they are knowledgeable in drug interactions and medical conditions, as well as in the homeopathic treatments appropriate to your condition.

Homeopathic remedies come in pellet, tablet, and liquid form. The liquid or mother tincture is an alcohol extract of a specific remedy. The liquid is generally placed under the tongue with an eyedropper that usually comes with it. Creams, ointments, or salves can be prepared by mixing the liquid with a cream or gel base. The creams and ointments are useful for sore muscles of the face and neck associated with temporomandibular joint disorders (TMJ) or long dental treatments. The tablets and pellets, which are made with a base of lactose (sweet milk sugar), are dissolved in the mouth, without chewing. These are excellent for children. Avoid touching them, as this may decrease their effectiveness. For infants, dissolve the pellet or tablet in water and give it to the child with an eyedropper. Since the liquid remedies contain alcohol, they should not be given to children.

It is advisable to take homeopathic treatments fifteen minutes before or after eating. Strong flavors such as mint and camphor, odors from perfumes and paints, and caffeine may decrease the effectiveness of the remedies.

Homeopathy requires personal observation to determine the length of treatment needed with each remedy. If no change occurs in a chronic ailment after a week, switch to another remedy. If improvement is noted, continue with the remedy until all symptoms have disappeared. If a new set of symptoms appears, start a different remedy.

COMMON HOMEOPATHIC THERAPEUTIC AGENTS

Agent	Indications
Acidum nitricum	Diarrhea caused by antibiotics.
Aconite	Anxiety, nervousness, fear, physical and mental restlessness, stiff and painful neck.
Ambra grisia	Children with extreme nervousness.
Ammonium carbonica	Pain on chewing, TMJ.
Ammonium phosphoricum	Facial paralysis.
Antimonium crudum	Dry lips, cracks at corners of lips, canker sores.
Antimonium tartaricum	Mouth sores caused by *Candida albicans*.
Apis mellifica	Swollen gums; red, sore tongue and throat; cancer of the tongue.
Arnica	Easily bleeding gums; dry, ulcerated tissues; dry, red tongue; toothache that is worse at night; metallic taste; sore muscles; pain, sprains.
Arsenicum album	Gums that bleed easily; dry mouth with ulcerations; dry, red, ulcerated tongue; neuralgia of teeth that is worse at night; metallic taste.
Arsenicum metallicum	Tongue that is coated white and shows imprint of teeth, ulcers in mouth.
Arum triphyllum	Cracked and sore corners of mouth.
Belladonna	Toothache, abscess, grinding of teeth, fever.
Bismuthum	Toothache that feels better with cold water, swollen gums.
Borax	Canker sores, bitter taste in mouth, dry mouth.
Bryonia	Cracked and dry lips, yellow- to dark brown-coated tongue.
Calcarea carbonica	Crackling noise and throbbing in ears, pulsating pain in teeth, swollen submaxillary glands, bleeding gums, toothache from hot or cold food or drinks, bad breath.
Calcarea fluorica	Loose teeth with toothache when chewing, oral tumors, teething pain.
Calendula	Cuts and other wounds caused by tooth extraction.
Capsicum	Oral herpes, bad breath.
Causticum	Facial paralysis, pain in facial bones, pain in jaws with difficulty in opening mouth.
Chamomilla	Toothache that intensifies with hot or warm foods or drinks, teething pain.
Dulcamara	Cold sores, especially on lips; symptoms of neuralgia.
Echinacea rudbeckia	Canker sores, receded gums that bleed easily, cracks at corners of lips, dry or swollen tongue.
Eupatorium perfoliatum	Cracks in corners of mouth, yellow-coated tongue, thirst.
Formalin	Loss of taste.
Gelsemium	Anxiety.
Hepar sulphuris	Painful, bleeding gums; depression; anxiety; swelling; infection; pain in jaw upon opening.
Hypericum	Injuries to nerves as in deep cavities; for pain control after any major dental treatment.
Ignatia	Mouth constantly full of saliva, toothache, sour taste.
Kali muriaticum	Pyorrhea, cold sores, thrush, swollen glands in neck and jaw.

Agent	Indications
Kali phosphoricum	Bad breath; excessive dry mouth in the morning; toothache; spongy, bleeding, and receding gums; anxiety.
Kreosotum	Children with anxiety.
Lachesis	Swollen, spongy, bleeding gums; cold sores; dry, cracked lips; pain in facial bones; lack of energy.
Lycopodium	Dry mouth, bad breath.
Magnesia phosphorica	Teething.
Magnesium carbonica	Toothache during pregnancy.
Mercurius corrosivus	Advanced gum disease with loose teeth and swollen, inflamed gums.
Mercurius cyanatus	Ulcerated mouth, pain and swelling of salivary glands.
Mercurius hydrargyrum	Gum disease, sore tongue.
Mercurius solubilis	Bad breath, excessive salivation, oral herpes. (Recommended during and after removal of many mercury fillings).
Mercurius vivus	Metallic-tasting saliva, bad breath, swollen gums, general body weakness.
Natrum muriaticum	Thick coating on tongue; numbness, tingling of tongue and lips; dry mouth; cracks at corners of mouth; loss of taste; unquenchable thirst.
Natrum phosphoricum	Canker sores on lips and cheeks.
Nux vomica	Bad breath caused by gastric disturbances.
Phosphorus	Easily bleeding gums, persistent bleeding after tooth extraction.
Phytolacca	Teething pain, pain in the soft palate, swollen tonsils.
Plantago major	Toothache that is sensitive to touch, worse with cold.
Pulsatilla	Toothache, bad breath, alteration or loss of taste, salivary gland disorder.
Pyrogenium	Bad breath; red, dry, and cracked tongue; dry throat; bad taste.
Rhamnus californica	Muscular pain and swollen joints in jaw (TMJ), canker sore between gums and lips.
Rhus toxicodendron	Loose teeth, sore gums, red and cracked tongue, cold sores around mouth, pain in jaw joint.
Santoninum	Headache, bad breath, thirst, loss of appetite, grinding of teeth.
Silicea	Gums sensitive to cold, abscess.
Staphysagria	Toothache during menstruation, anger, mood swings.
Sulphur	Skin rash.
Sulphuricum acidum	Cold sores, gums that bleed easily, anxiety, craving for stimulants.
Symphytum	Anxiety after trauma.
Trillium pendulum	Excessive bleeding after tooth extraction, bleeding gums, headache in front of head.
Upas tiente	Herpes on lips.
Xerophyllum	Headache, backache, TMJ, pressure in sinuses and behind eyes.
X-ray	Excessive exposure to x-rays, painful throat when swallowing.

Herbal Therapy

An herb, botanically speaking, is any plant that lacks the woody tissue characteristic of shrubs or trees. More specifically, herbs are plants used medicinally or for their flavor or scent. Herbs with medicinal properties are a useful and effective source of treatment for various disease processes. Many drugs used in Western medical science—called allopathic medicine—have their origin in medicinal plants.

In 2735 B.C., a Chinese emperor recommended an extract from the *ma huang* plant (known as *ephedra* in the Western world) as a treatment for respiratory illness. Today, the chemical ephedrine is extracted from the plant and used as a decongestant (e.g., pseudoephedrine). Codeine, derived from opium, has long been used as an analgesic and cough suppressant.

During the Golden Age of Western herbology, which occurred from 500 B.C. to 200 A.D., Western physicians and scholars classified hundreds of plants useful in healing. By the Middle Ages, every household had an herb garden to supply it with medicines. Rhubarb was used as a laxative. Salicin, a forerunner of aspirin (acetylsalicylic acid), was derived from the bark of the willow tree. The tranquilizer laudanum, derived from the poppy, was later used to treat the "vapors" experienced by Victorian ladies.

By World War II, herbology was losing popularity in the West. Penicillin and other "wonder drugs" seemed to be cure-alls. And the war itself had cut off supplies of herbs from around the world. The advent of the drug industry with its synthetic medicines seemed to ring a death knoll for herbology, yet plants remain a major source of drugs today. For example, the previously mentioned ephedrine, digitalis (a heart strengthener), and vincristine (an antitumor drug) are all plant-derived.

Ironically, the same research that threatened to make herbal medicine extinct has also proven its efficacy, breathing new life into it. We now know that the peppermint used for digestive disorders since 1800 B.C. relieves nausea and vomiting by mildly anesthetizing the stomach lining. Laboratory analysis has shown that herbs contain vital vitamins, minerals, and natural chemicals that may be essential to curing a diseased body. Echinacea, for instance, is derived from the purple coneflower and was used by herbalists for centuries to fight infection. Research has shown that echinacea stimulates the production of white blood cells, thereby boosting the immune system.

Many moderns, in support of herbal therapies, believe that extracting the chemical rather than using the whole plant eliminates such active ingredients as minerals, volatile oils, bioflavonoids, and other substances that support a particular herb's medicinal properties. Some feel that isolated or synthesized compounds may have harmful side effects because they are so concentrated.

Generally speaking, herbs are used to cleanse the blood, warm and stimulate the body, increase surface circulation, increase elimination of wastes, reduce inflammation, and calm and soothe irritation. Herbs may be used internally as pills, syrups, and infusions, or externally as poultices, plasters, and liniments. An external application of clove oil, for instance, will stop the pain of toothache, as will tincture of hops. Herbs are commonly used as additives to bath water—either full body baths or baths for the foot, eye, or face. Moist herbal wraps, either hot or cold, can be used on specific affected parts of the body. These wraps are especially effective for sore, tense muscles such as those in the neck, shoulders, back, or jaw when temporomandibular joint syndrome (TMJ) is present.

Herbs, which are powerful healing agents, must be used appropriately. Always know what you are taking. Keep in mind that not all plant life is beneficial. Certain herbs may be toxic, especially when used over a long period of time or in too great amounts. Herbs contain active ingredients that may interact negatively with prescribed medications or other remedies. It is wise, therefore, to consult a health-care professional in situations in which you question the appropriateness of the herb or its interaction with other remedies. Also note that the herbal recommendations found in Part Two are for adults, not children.

The herbs most commonly used for dental problems are described below. Specific advice on the use of these herbs for various conditions can be found in Part Two. Directions for preparing various herbal remedies can be found under Using Herbs in Part Three.

Alfalfa

Also known as buffalo herb, alfalfa grows in dry fields, in sandy wastes, and along some roadsides. It reaches a height of one to two feet and has bluish flowers from June through August. The leaves, petals, flowers, and sprouts are commonly used to treat stomach and blood disorders. One of the richest sources of trace minerals and an antioxidant, alfalfa is high in calcium, iron, magnesium, phosphorus, potassium, chlorine, and vitamin K.

Precautions and Recommendations

- Alfalfa is useful in cases of hemorrhaging and fungal infections.
- Available in liquid form, it is an excellent choice as a mineral supplement.

Aloe Vera

A native of southern Africa, the aloe vera plant has fleshy spiny-toothed leaves and red or yellow flowers. It is an ingredient in many cosmetics because it heals, moisturizes, and softens skin. Simply cut one of the aloe vera leaves to easily extract the soothing gel.

Precautions and Recommendations

- Aloe vera gel should not be taken internally in large quantities by those who have hemorrhoids or an irritated colon.

- Pregnant women should not take aloe internally.
- Applied externally, aloe vera gel is excellent for soothing inflamed gums and sores in the mouth.

Anise

Also known as sweet fennel, anise is a native of Egypt. It grows to a height of ten or twelve inches and has light green leaves and small yellow-white flowers. The licorice-flavored seeds are used in medicine and as a flavoring.

Precautions and Recommendations

- An anti-inflammatory herb, anise is commonly used in tea form to soothe the gums.
- Chew fennel seeds whole to eliminate bad breath.

Annatto

A small tropical American tree, annatto is a rich source of vitamins A and D—richer than cod-liver oil. The pulp of the seeds, which is used in cooking, yields a yellowish-red dye. The pulp is also used medicinally.

Precautions and Recommendations

- Apply annatto after tooth extraction or gum surgery.

Arnica

A mountain plant that grows to about twenty inches in height, arnica has yellow-orange flowers that bloom in the summer. Arnica flowers are commonly used to combat fever, and to stimulate the heart, circulation, and digestive system. Arnica is also a homeopathic remedy.

Precautions and Recommendations

- Available in creams and ointments, arnica can be externally applied to relieve bruises, strains, sprains, pain, and muscle tension.

Bee Pollen

Fresh pollen obtained from bees contains amino acids, calcium, carotene, copper, enzymes, iron, magnesium, manganese, potassium, B vitamins, vitamin C, and other chemicals and nutrients. It is effective for combating fatigue, depression, and colon disorders. Pollen has an antimicrobial effect.

Precautions and Recommendations

- A small percentage of the population is allergic to bee pollen. Use with caution, starting with small amounts and discontinuing if a rash, wheezing, or other symptoms develop.

Black Cohosh

This tall plant, native to eastern North America, has long clusters of small white flowers. Its rhizomes and roots contain estrogenic substances, phosphorus, vitamins A and B5, and several other chemicals and nutrients. Black cohosh is commonly used to treat pain and reduce mucus levels.

Precautions and Recommendations

- Do not take black cohosh if you are pregnant or have a chronic disease.
- Overdoses will cause nausea and vomiting.
- Use black cohosh to relieve cramps in the jaw or neck.

Burdock

A common plant that grows in almost any moist soil, burdock grows from two to six feet high and has burs. The very large leaves—up to two feet long—are poisonous.

Burdock is considered an excellent blood purifier. Its roots and seeds contain a variety of chemicals and nutrients, including biotin, copper, iron, manganese, sulfur, zinc, and vitamins B1, B6, B12, and E. These plant parts are commonly used to treat skin disorders and stimulate the immune system.

Precautions and Recommendations

- Taken internally, burdock root interferes with iron absorption.
- Burdock poultices (see Using Herbs, Application Preparation, in Part Three) are excellent for the relief of muscle tension and headaches associated with temporomandibular joint disorders (TMJ).

Catnip

A common wild plant, catnip may reach three feet in height. Its leaves are long with downy undersides, and it has clusters of pale pink, spotted flowers. The leaves have traditionally been used to treat the nerves and intestines. Catnip is excellent for calming the nervous system and controlling irritability. It contains many chemicals and nutrients, including acetic acid, manganese, phosphorus, PABA, sodium, sulfur, vitamin A, and several B vitamins.

Precautions and Recommendations

- Drink catnip tea or take in capsules to help you relax before dental treatment. (See Using Herbs, Tea Preparation, in Part Three.)

Cayenne

The pungent fruit of the *Capsicum frutescens*, cayenne is used to treat the heart, circulation, stomach, and kidneys. Cayenne stops both internal and external bleeding.

Precautions and Recommendations

- When cooked, cayenne becomes an irritant.
- Saturate cotton with oil of cayenne and place it on an aching tooth for emergency relief.

Chamomile

Chamomile grows in well-drained sunny soil in temperate regions everywhere. A hardy perennial that reaches a height of one foot, chamomile has daisylike blossoms. Commonly used as a nerve tonic, sleep aid, and digestive aid, chamomile is also a homeopathic remedy. It contains calcium, iron, magnesium, manganese, potassium, and vitamin A.

Precautions and Recommendations

- Use chamomile as a poultice for pain and swelling. (See Using Herbs, Application Preparation, in Part Three.)
- Drink as a hot tea to promote relaxation. (See Using Herbs, Tea Preparation, in Part Three.)
- Use as a mouthwash to soothe inflamed, irritated gums. (See Using Herbs, Mouthwash Preparation, in Part Three.)

Chickweed

The most common of weeds, chickweed is found throughout the world. Its leaves are used to soothe skin irritations.

Precautions and Recommendations

- Chickweed mouthwash soothes inflamed, irritated mouth tissues associated with oral cancer; it also helps to relieve pain from canker sores and other mouth sores. (See Using Herbs, Mouthwash Preparation, in Part Three.)

Cloves

The dried flower buds of an East Indian evergreen tree, cloves are popularly used as a spice. They also yield a volatile oil used medicinally and in perfumes. Cloves have antiseptic, stimulant, and antiemetic (vomiting preventive) properties and are used to treat the mouth, stomach, intestines, circulation, and lungs.

Precautions and Recommendations

- Rub oil of cloves on sore gums and teeth to ease pain.
- Chew whole cloves to diminish bad breath.

Comfrey

The comfrey plant grows in rich, moist areas and has prickly green leaves along its stalk, which can reach three feet in height. White flowers bloom at the top of the comfrey plant. Its leaves and roots have traditionally been used to treat the lungs, stomach, and intestines. Comfrey contains phosphorus, potassium, starch, tannins, and vitamins A, C, and E.

Precautions and Recommendations

- Do not use comfrey for longer than three months at a time as it may cause liver damage.
- Soak a washcloth in warm comfrey tea and use as a compress (see Using Herbs, Application Preparation, in Part Three) to ease jaw tension and relieve the pain of jaw and tooth fractures or adjustments to braces.

Dandelion

Commonly thought of as a weed, the dandelion flowers from April to November. It has long been used to make tea and wine and is a popular seasoning in old English recipes. The leaves, roots, and tops are used to treat a variety of internal organs and to purify blood. It also increases the production of bile and urine. Dandelion contains biotin, calcium, choline, fats, iron, magnesium, niacin, PABA, phosphorus, proteins, sulfur, zinc, and a variety of vitamins.

Precautions and Recommendations

- Dandelion is useful for treating abscesses in the mouth.
- Use as a blood purifier.

Echinacea

Historically used against syphilis and gonorrhea, echinacea is a good blood cleanser. Its roots and leaves contain many enzymes, fatty acids, and polysaccharides, which are recognized as immune system stimulators. The plants also contain copper, glucose, iron, potassium, protein, sucrose, sulfur, and vitamins A, C, and E. Echinacea has antibiotic, antiviral, and anti-inflammatory properties.

Precautions and Recommendations

- The alcohol used to prepare tinctures may destroy echinacea's polysaccharides. The freeze-dried form is preferred.
- Combined with myrrh and licorice root, echinacea is excellent for the treatment of abscesses in the mouth.

Elderberry

The small edible fruit of the elder—a plant that can reach twelve feet and grows in damp ground—elderberries are a rich source of vitamin C. The dark purple berries are often used to make wine or preserves and have traditionally been used to treat colic, diarrhea, rheumatism, coughs, and colds.

Precautions and Recommendations

- Prepare elderberry mouthwash (see Using Herbs, Mouthwash Preparation, in Part Three) after gum surgery or after sutures have been placed. The rinse will help tissues to heal properly, thereby preventing scars.

Eucalyptus

A tall tree native to Australia, the eucalyptus yields a powerfully antiseptic essential oil that has long been used medicinally. As its leaves have commonly been used to lower fevers, the eucalyptus is sometimes known as the "fever tree."

Precautions and Recommendations

- Rub eucalyptus oil on sore, inflamed gums for temporary relief.

Evening Primrose

The evening primrose, a native of North America, has four-petaled yellow flowers that open in the evening. The seeds yield an oil that contains gamma-linolenic acid, linoleic acid, and vitamin F. Evening primrose oil is used to treat skin disorders, arthritis, alcoholism, and other disorders. It also aids in weight loss and in reducing high blood pressure.

Precautions and Recommendations

- Rub evening primrose oil on sore, inflamed gums for temporary relief.

Fennel

See Anise.

Garlic

A plant related to the onion, garlic has a bulb that is divided into cloves. Garlic has been used for centuries to prevent and treat a variety of illnesses and to ensure longevity. Today, it is used as a natural antibiotic that is good for fighting infections caused by fungi or bacteria. It helps strengthen the immune system and is used to lower blood pressure. Garlic is also used to treat arteriosclerosis, asthma, arthritis, and digestive and circulatory problems. Garlic contains calcium, copper, germanium, iron, magnesium, manganese, phosphorus, vitamins A, B_1, B_2, and C, and a variety of other chemicals.

Precautions and Recommendations

- Fresh oil of garlic or raw cloves are considered the most effective forms.
- Odorless garlic extract, sold in health-food stores under the name Kyolic, is available.

Gentian

Gentian root (*Gentiana lutea*) is a powerful stimulant that is effective for such conditions as poor appetite and slow digestive system. Taken as a powerful tonic, gentian helps purify the blood and enhance circulation. It is also effective in fever reduction.

Precautions and Recommendations

- Those with high blood pressure and pregnant women should not take gentian.
- The usual dose of gentian is 1 to 30 grams before meals. Overdose can cause nausea and vomiting.

Ginseng

There are two varieties of ginseng, one native to eastern Asia and the other native to North America. Both have small greenish flowers and a forked root. It is the root that has medicinal properties. Like the famous mandrake root, the ginseng root is shaped like a man. In China at one time, the ginseng root was believed to have almost magical qualities and was used in such quantity that it became nearly extinct. At that time, the Chinese began to import American ginseng, which is now grown commercially.

The ginseng root is used as a whole-body tonic. It promotes appetite and is used for digestive disturbances and in cases of impotence. It contains calcium, camphor, iron, starch, and vitamins A, B_{12}, and E, along with other chemicals.

Precautions and Recommendations

- Large amounts of ginseng should not be used by elderly or weak people who have high fevers.
- Use in a tonic to promote circulation and to help repair irritated gum tissue.

Glucomannan

Derived from the tuber amorphophallis plant, glucomannan helps regulate blood glucose levels and aids in the removal of toxins from the colon.

Precautions and Recommendations

- Take glucomannan to eliminate toxic substances produced during digestion.
- Do not take glucomannan along with any medications or supplements. This may interfere with the effectiveness of glucomannan's fiber substances.

Goldenseal

Once, this herb grew wild in the woods of eastern North America. Now, the wild form is almost extinct, but goldenseal is cultivated in shady areas with rich soil.

The yellow root-stalk has large rounded leaves. The roots and rhizomes have been popular as both internal and external remedies. Internally, they are used for all problems involving mucous membranes. Externally, they are used to help relieve open sores, inflammations, and itchy skin conditions. Goldenseal has anti-inflammatory and antibacterial properties. It contains biotin, calcium, chlorine, choline, fats, iron, manganese, PABA, phosphorus, potassium, starch, the B-complex vitamins, and vitamins A, C, and E.

Precautions and Recommendations

- Long-term use of goldenseal may reduce the bacterial flora in the colon.

- When used as a toothpaste or mouthwash, goldenseal is excellent for soothing inflamed gums. (See Using Herbs, Toothpaste Preparation and Mouthwash Preparation, in Part Three.)

Hops

Native to northern temperate zones, hops are grown commercially for use in beer, bitters, and ales. Hops vines grow to eighteen feet and have conelike flowers and seedlike fruits. The leaves have three to five lobes and are deep green and very rough. The fruits and leaves are used to treat nervousness, stress, and pain. Among the chemicals and nutrients contained in hops are choline, manganese, PABA, and vitamin B_6.

Precautions and Recommendations

- Prepare hops tea (see Using Herbs, Tea Preparation, in Part Three) and drink as a remedy for toothache.

- Drink hops tea to promote sleep and relaxation.

Horsetail

The prehistoric horsetail plant is rich in healing silica and is commonly used to reduce fever. It also has anti-inflammatory properties, stops bleeding, and repairs damaged tissue.

Precautions and Recommendations

- Use a horsetail mouthwash to relieve mouth and gum infections. (See Using Herbs, Mouthwash Preparation, in Part Three.)

Kelp

A large brown seaweed, kelp contains biotin, bromine, calcium, choline, copper, iodine, PABA, potassium, a variety of B vitamins, vitamins C and E, and other chemicals and nutrients. It is used to treat the sensory nerves, goiter, ulcers, and obesity, and to protect people against the effects of radiation. Kelp is available in tablet or powder form.

Precautions and Recommendations

- One of the richest sources of vitamins, minerals, and trace elements, kelp taken daily will help ensure healthy gums and bone.

Licorice Root

Often called "the grandfather of herbs," licorice root has been used medicinally for thousands of years. Beneficial as an anti-inflammatory for arthritic or allergic conditions, licorice root is also used as a digestive stimulant and a soothing expectorant for lung disorders, such as asthma and bronchitis. Its antibiotic properties are effective in the treatment of ulcers. There is further evidence that glycyrrhizin, the active ingredient in licorice, inhibits plaque growth and is effective against *Streptococcus mutans*, the bacteria associated with tooth cavity development. Sweet and flavorful, licorice is often added to toothpaste and mouthwash.

Precautions and Recommendations

- Drink licorice tea to promote a healthy immune system. (See Using Herbs, Tea Preparation, in Part Three.)

- Do not take licorice if you have high blood pressure, heart problems, or if you are taking digoxin-based drugs.

Lobelia

In the wild, lobelia is a small weed that grows abundantly in the eastern United States. The plant and its seeds have traditionally been used to treat the lungs, stomach, muscles, and circulatory system. Recently, an alkaloid in the plant (lobeline) has been used as an aid in breaking the smoking habit. In addition to the alkaloids, lobelia contains chelidonic acid, selenium, and sulfur. Lobelia aids in hormone production; it is also used as a cough suppressant and powerful relaxant.

Precautions and Recommendations

- Mix lobelia with black cohosh, skullcap, cayenne, and myrrh, and prepare as a tea. (See Using Herbs, Tea Preparation, in Part Three.) Drink to ease jaw pain.

Marigold

An annual herb that grows to two feet in height, the marigold has a "hairy" stem and leaves. The flowers are yellow or orange-yellow, and the fruit is semicircular with a strong, unpleasant odor. Commonly used as a homeopathic remedy (*Calendula*, called "the homeopathic antiseptic"), marigold flowers have been used internally as a diuretic, a stimulant, and an antispasmodic. Externally, they are used in the treatment of burns, wounds, and impetigo of the scalp.

Precautions and Recommendations

- Use marigold as a mouthwash (see Using Herbs, Mouthwash Preparation, in Part Three) to help relieve ulcers, wounds, or inflamed areas, and to relax muscles associated with tension in the jaw joint and pressure from braces.

Marjoram

Marjoram, either sweet or wild, grows in dry pastures and at the edges of woodlands. The plants of either variety grow to approximately twenty feet, and have a pyramidal shape, faded and aromatic rose-colored flowers, and leaves with downy undersides. The flowering tips are used to flavor foods and prepare home remedies. In ancient times, marjoram was used to combat acidity and flatulence. Today, it is considered an antispasmodic, expectorant, antiseptic, and stomachic.

Precautions and Recommendations

- Prepare marjoram as tea (see Using Herbs, Tea Preparation, in Part Three). Drink hot to ease headaches and relieve toothache pain.

Myrrh

A gum obtained from the trees and shrubs of the genus *Commiphora*, myrrh may be best known as one of the gifts the Wise Men brought to the Infant Jesus. Myrrh is a powerful antiseptic that has long been used to treat stomach and lung disorders.

Precautions and Recommendations

- Taken in large quantities or over a long period of time, myrrh can be toxic.
- Myrrh helps promote healing in cases of pyorrhea. Rinse the mouth with myrrh tea and brush with the powder when gum disease exists. (See Using Herbs, Tea Preparation, in Part Three.)
- Gargle with myrrh to help eliminate bad breath. (See Using Herbs, Mouthwash Preparation, in Part Three.)

Parsley

An aromatic herb commonly used as a garnish or seasoning for food, parsley contains potassium and vitamins A and C. It is also a natural diuretic.

Precautions and Recommendations

- Chewing on a sprig of sweet, aromatic parsley will help eliminate bad breath.
- Excessive amounts of parsley may stop milk production in nursing mothers.

Peppermint

This mint grows in moist, open areas to a height of three feet and has dark green, lance-shaped leaves and purple flowers. One of the oldest of household remedies, it has been used to treat the stomach, intestines, and muscles, and to improve circulation. The leaves and flowering tops are now used to treat colic, fever, convulsions, and especially nausea and diarrhea. Peppermint contains menthol, methyl acetate, tannic acid, and vitamin C.

Precautions and Recommendations

- Peppermint may interfere with iron absorption.
- Use peppermint oil for toothache. Soak a cotton ball in the oil and place it in the cavity or rub it on the tooth.
- Use peppermint mouthwash to relieve gum inflammation. (See Using Herbs, Mouthwash Preparation, in Part Three.)

Prickly Ash

An aromatic shrub or small tree native to eastern North America, the prickly ash has prickly stems and feathery leaves. The bark has traditionally been used to treat the circulatory and digestive systems. Powdered bark is used as a poultice for wounds.

Precautions and Recommendations

- If taken when the stomach is irritable, prickly ash may cause vomiting.
- Use to increase the flow of saliva.

Red Clover

Used mainly as a blood purifier, the blossoms of the red clover are also helpful in treating acne, boils, and skin infections. It is also effective as a mild sedative.

Precautions and Recommendations

- For a general calming effect, drink warm red clover tea. (See Using Herbs, Tea Preparation, in Part Three.)
- Red clover mouthwash is healing for irritated, diseased gums. (See Using Herbs, Mouthwash Preparation, in Part Three.)
- After making red clover tea, prepare an ointment from the strained blossoms and leaves. (See Using Herbs, Application Preparation, in Part Three.) Rub the ointment, which has antibiotic properties, on gums that are abscessed from disease, or sore and inflamed from root canal therapy or other dental procedures.

Rockrose

Sometimes referred to as sun rose, this low-growing evergreen of the genus *Helianthemum* loves the sun. It is helpful in reducing anxiety.

Precautions and Recommendations

- Use rockrose mouthwash to soothe and heal canker sores and mouth ulcers. (See Using Herbs, Mouthwash Preparation, in Part Three.)
- Drink rockrose tea to promote relaxation. (See Using Herbs, Tea Preparation, in Part Three.)

Rosemary

Native to the Mediterranean region, this evergreen shrub is widely grown for its aromatic leaves, which are used as a seasoning, in perfume, and for medicinal purposes. Long used to treat the stomach, intestines, liver, nerves, and lungs, rosemary increases the production of bile and raises blood pressure.

Precautions and Recommendations

- Drink rosemary tea as a stimulant (see Using Herbs, Tea Preparation, in Part Three); do not drink more than three cups a day.
- Use rosemary mouthwash for the treatment of gum disease and bad breath. (See Using Herbs, Mouthwash Preparation, in Part Three.)

Sage

A member of the mint family, sage grows wild in fields and along roadsides. The plants have square stems that grow to eighteen inches in height. From May to June, the grayish-green evergreen leaves are accompanied by purple flowers. Revered by the Romans as a giver of life, sage was an obligatory ingredient in medicinal preparations during the Middle Ages. Today, the leaves are used to treat laryngitis, tonsillitis, and sore throats. The herb also has antiflatulent and mildly laxative properties.

Precautions and Recommendations

- Lactating women should not drink sage tea; it can interfere with production of breast milk.
- As a mild antiseptic, this herb will help heal bleeding gums and mouth ulcers (cold sores).
- Drink a cup of hot sage and chamomile tea to ease apprehension before dental treatment. (See Using Herbs, Tea Preparation, in Part Three.)

Sanicle

A perennial that grows to two feet in height, sanicle has finely toothed leaves and pale flowers. The seeds are contained in round burs. This herb was used long ago to dissipate "evil humours," and was considered a panacea. Today, the flowering tips and leaves—rich in tannin, resin, and essential oil—are used for their antiseptic, anti-inflammatory, stomachic, and astringent properties.

Precautions and Recommendations

- Use sanicle when a powerful antioxidant is desired.
- Use as a salve or ointment to heal septic wounds. (See Using Herbs, Application Preparation, in Part Three.)

Sarsaparilla

A perennial climber with prickly stems, sarsaparilla has large leaves, red or black berries, and yellowish flowers that bloom from late spring to late summer. It was once considered an antidote against all venemous things. The roots—which contain hormones, iron, manganese, sodium, sulfur, vitamins A and D, and zinc—are now used to treat skin eruptions and arthritic conditions. Sarsaparilla tea increases the flow of urine, breaks up gas, and is a good eyewash.

Precautions and Recommendations

- Drink sarsaparilla tea to promote relaxation and to protect against harmful radiation. (See Using Herbs, Tea Preparation, in Part Three).

Shepherd's Purse

Also known as St. John's wort, shepherd's purse is a very common "weed" that grows to about eighteen inches in height and has tiny white flowers. The tops are used for their astringent, diuretic, and stimulant properties. As a homeopathic remedy, it is known as *Hypericum*.

Precautions and Recommendations

- Use the fresh tops of shepherd's purse to help stop bleeding after tooth extraction.

Skullcap

An herb with clusters of two-lipped flowers, skullcap is used to treat nervous disorders, migraine headaches, rheumatism, and convulsions. It contains glycoside, iron, sugar, tannins, and vitamin E. Skullcap's aerial parts (leaves) help relieve pain, stress, cramps, and spasms, as well as improve circulation.

Precautions and Recommendations

- Drink skullcap tea to relieve anxiety before a dental appointment. (See Using Herbs, Tea Preparation, in Part Three.)

Summer Savory

A hardy annual, summer savory grows to eight or nine inches in height and has small stringy roots, "hairy" branches, and white flowers tinged with pink or lilac. Commonly used as an aromatic herb in cooking, summer savory has therapeutic properties, particularly for the stomach and bowels. The dried tops are used to treat colic, flatulence, diarrhea, poor digestion, and frayed nerves.

Precautions and Recommendations

- Soak a cotton ball with summer savory oil and place it on a sore tooth or rub it on inflamed gums for temporary relief.

- Drink summer savory tea to promote relaxation. (See Using Herbs, Tea Preparation, in Part Three.)

Tea Tree Oil

Derived from the Australian malaluca tree, tea tree oil is used in several commercial products including mouthwash and toothpaste. It is highly antiseptic and antifungal for cuts and abrasions, as well as warts and cold sores.

Precautions and Recommendations

- Rub tea tree oil directly on cold sores to promote healing. (Apply to the area as soon as a developing cold sore starts to tingle.)

- Rub tea tree oil directly on sore, inflamed gums for temporary relief.

- Use tea tree oil mouthwash to soothe mouth inflammation. (See Using Herbs, Mouthwash Preparation, in Part Three.)

Thyme

A member of the mint family, thyme grows wild in moist fields and along roadsides. It has a square, slim, woody stem that reaches about a foot in height, small leaves, and a pungent aroma. Thyme has been used since ancient times to, among other things, embalm the dead and enhance beauty. It is a powerful antiseptic (bacilli exposed to thyme essence do not survive for more than forty minutes), and the leaves and flowers are used to treat chronic respiratory problems, colds, sore throats, and the flu. Thyme contains fluorine, trace minerals, thiamine, thymol, the B-complex vitamins, and vitamins C and D.

Precautions and Recommendations

- Use a salve made of thyme, myrrh, and goldenseal to treat oral herpes. (See Using Herbs, Application Preparation, in Part Three.)
- As thyme is a uterine stimulant, therapeutic doses in any form should be avoided by pregnant women.

Violet

Violets (*Clematis virginica*) have been used medicinally since ancient times. Known for their sedative properties, violets are also used for a wide range of skin disorders.

Precautions and Recommendations

- Mouthwash made from violets helps relieve the pain and tenderness from sores caused by oral cancer. It is also helpful in soothing canker sores and cold sores. (See Using Herbs, Mouthwash Preparation, in Part Three.)

Wintergreen

A perennial that grows in fertile forest areas with other evergreens, wintergreen has a creeping root, grows to about ten inches in height, and produces a spike of white flowers. The leaves have long been used to treat wounds and stop hemorrhages. Today, wintergreen is considered a good remedy for cystitis because it flushes the urinary tract and contains a natural antiseptic.

Precautions and Recommendations

- Wintergreen mouthwash is an excellent astringent and antiseptic. (See Using Herbs, Mouthwash Preparation, in Part Three.)
- Soak a cotton ball in wintergreen oil and place it on a sore tooth or rub it on inflamed gums for temporary relief.

Witch Hazel

A shrub native to eastern North America, witch hazel has yellow flowers that bloom in late autumn. The bark and leaves have astringent, sedative, and hemostatic (acting to stop the flow of blood) properties. Witch hazel is used internally to treat excessive blood flow during menstruation and hemorrhages. Externally, it is good for healing sores and wounds.

Precautions and Recommendations

- Use witch hazel mouthwash to cleanse the mouth and help fight infections. (See Using Herbs, Mouthwash Preparation, in Part Three.)

Wood Betony

Also known as lousewort, wood betony grows in shady places and reaches heights of twelve to twenty-three inches. The stem is slightly hairy with aromatic leaves and purplish flowers arranged in terminal spikes. In ancient times, wood betony was considered the "infallible remedy" for almost fifty serious diseases, including rabies. Today, the leaves are used to treat diseases that stem from impurities of the blood, to kill intestinal worms, and to heal open wounds. Wood betony contains magnesium, manganese, phosphorus, and tannins.

Precautions and Recommendations

- Drink wood betony tea to promote relaxation before a dental appointment. (See Using Herbs, Tea Preparation, in Part Three.)

Yarrow

The yarrow plant grows in pastures, in meadows, and along roadsides. It stands ten to twenty inches tall and has many downy, toothed leaves, white or pale rose flowers, and oblong fruit. Achilles is said to have been the first to use yarrow to cure wounds; hence its scientific name *Achillea millefolium*. The leaves and fruits are now used to treat hemorrhages, ulcers, and chicken pox, and to heal mucous membranes, ease diarrhea, and improve blood clotting. Yarrow contains potassium, tannins, and vitamin C, as well as other chemicals and nutrients.

Precautions and Recommendations

- Yarrow interferes with absorption of iron and other minerals.
- Use yarrow mouthwash to promote healing of cuts in mouth due to surgery, teeth cleaning, and braces. (See Using Herbs, Mouthwash Preparation, in Part Three.)

Choosing a Dentist

There are many factors to consider when choosing a dentist or, for that matter, any practitioner. One major factor should be the dentist's ability to perform techniques properly. Ability may be influenced by the dentist's educational background and number of years in practice. Other common factors to consider include the dentist's attitude or level of caring for your condition, cost of treatment, and, last but not least, the appearance of the office or place where the treatment is rendered—are the surroundings clean? Do you feel comfortable there?

In choosing a dentist, you will need to answer the following questions:

HOW DO I BEGIN LOOKING FOR THE RIGHT DENTIST?

Getting referrals from friends or family members is a good way to start looking for a dentist. If you have no personal referrals, you can also get names from a dental referral service, such as 1-800-DENTIST or 1-800-DEN-TAL-911. Be aware, however, that such services are nothing more than fee-for-service agencies. The dentist pays a monthly fee to the agency, who in turn, provides interested callers with general information about the dentist and his or her practice. Such information includes the dentist's educational background and years in practice, as well as the office location. Local dental societies and hospitals also provide referrals, but like the agencies, they offer only general information about the dentist. The last place you should look for a dentist is in the *Yellow Pages*, which provides nothing more than a list of licensed practitioners.

When calling different dental offices, be sure to have a list of questions on hand, such as treatment costs, insurance procedures, emergency-care availability, office hours, staff size, and available diagnostic techniques and safety devices (e.g. sterilization techniques, protection devices for x-ray radiation). When you first call an office, you will likely speak to a receptionist, who should be equipped to answer any general questions. (Dentists themselves generally do not have the time to talk with you by phone, especially if you are not already a patient.) Specific questions about your particular dental needs, however, cannot be answered until you are seen by the dentist. Most dental offices will let you set up an appointment for a short "interview" with the dentist before actually committing to treatment. During this interview you will be able to evaluate the office and see if you feel comfortable with the dentist. Unlike a "consultation"—for which there is usually a fee— an interview does not give you the opportunity to ask questions about your specific dental needs.

WHAT TRAINING HAS THE DENTIST HAD?

At least two years of college education are required before admission to dental schools; however, most dental students are college graduates. The programs provided at American dental schools are fairly similar to each other. Most schools offer a four-year course of study. The first two years involve basic medical and dental sciences as well as dental laboratory techniques, while the last two years emphasize clinical aspects of dentistry (treating patients). Once dental school is completed, students receive either a Doctor of Dental Surgery (D.D.S.) degree or a Doctor of Dental Medicine (D.M.D.) degree. There is no difference between the two degrees; some colleges call it the former and others call it the latter. Dentists who earned their degrees in foreign countries must complete a year or more of training in an accredited dental school in order to practice in the United States.

Dentists wishing to specialize in a field need one to four additional years of training, after which they are considered specialists in that field. They are then qualified to take a board exam in that specialty and become board certified by their particular specialty group. A dentist may also receive an additional honorary title that entitles him or her to be referred to as a "fellow" of a particular group. The title "fellow" can also be obtained by a dentist who completes certain continuing education courses or becomes a member of a group. For example, members of the Academy of General Dentistry are given a certificate entitling them to use FAGD (Fellow of the Academy of General Dentistry) after their names.

WHAT KIND OF DENTIST DO I NEED?

General dentistry involves all aspects of dentistry. The general practitioner provides treatments that include filling cavities, cleaning teeth, extracting teeth, and replacing lost teeth. The general dentist may employ a dental hygienist to clean teeth. A dental hygienist must complete a two-year program of study to be certified as such.

Dentists who specialize in pediatric (children's) dentistry are called *pedodontists*. Some children may require special attention that only a pedodontist is trained to offer. *Endodontists* diagnose and treat diseased tooth pulp and perform root canal work. The replacement of missing or damaged teeth is performed by *prosthodontists*. A prosthodontist may specialize in either removable (dentures) or fixed (bridges) prosthetics. Prosthodontists may also perform procedures to improve the balance between the teeth, called occlusal equilibration. *Oral pathologists* use laboratory procedures to diagnose diseases of the mouth. The oral pathologist also specializes in forensic dentistry and identifies dead people by comparing their teeth with dental records. *Periodontists* treat diseases of the supporting structures of the teeth, including bone and gum tissue. *Oral surgeons* remove cysts, tumors, and wisdom teeth that may be too difficult for the general practitioner to remove. They also correct fractures or other jaw problems that require surgery. Cosmetic problems of the jaw and face are corrected by *maxillofacial surgeons* using methods similar to those of plastic surgery. Improperly positioned teeth are corrected by *orthodontists*.

Orthodontists use braces or other mechanical devices to move teeth into a better position.

IS THE DENTIST LICENSED?

Dentists must be licensed to practice. Once a D.D.S. or D.M.D. is obtained, a state and national exam must be passed before a license is granted. General practitioners as well as specialists are required to complete continuing education courses every two years in order to renew their licenses.

WHAT IS THE DENTIST'S ATTITUDE?

Choose a dentist who is willing to take the time to answer your questions. The purpose and goal of every dental practitioner should be to help you understand the cause of your problem so that you can prevent its recurrence, and to help you choose among treatment options. However, in our fast-paced society, where time means money, a great many practitioners are unlikely to spend time with you. Choose a practitioner who can balance time and money properly.

It is also very important for a practitioner, especially a dentist, to have a caring attitude about rendering treatment. Some people associate dental treatment with pain and fear. A dentist's ability to make you feel relaxed and confident in his or her treatment is certainly an important consideration.

After you read this book and increase your understanding of dentistry basics, you will be able to find a dentist with whom you can communicate and from whom you can get the best treatment for a reasonable cost.

Also consider the attitude of the office staff. Observe how well those who work in the office get along. Is everyone willing to help you, or are staff members busy performing too many tasks? A staff that sees fewer patients per hour has more time to devote to each patient than does the staff in an overly busy office.

ARE HEALTH AND SAFETY GUIDELINES FOLLOWED?

Office cleanliness is extremely important in these days of AIDS awareness. Due to the nature of dental treatment, many fear that AIDS may be transmitted during treatment. Proper sterilization techniques will help minimize the risk of disease transmission. Soaking instruments in a cold chemical solution is not an adequate means of destroying germs. There are several viable methods of ensuring that instruments are sterile. Use of disposable instruments is the most preferred method. The use of autoclaves, chemical vapor sterilizers, and dry heat sterilizers are others.

Autoclaves employ pressurized steam at a prescribed temperature. Similar to a pressure cooker, water is heated to boiling, steam is created, and the elevated temperature sterilizes the instruments. Chemical vapor sterilizers use a mixture of chemicals, including formaldehyde, alcohol, and acetone along with water. At high temperatures, the chemicals vaporize and sterilize the instruments that are placed in a chamber. Dry heat sterilizers utilize an electrical heating element capable of heating the chamber to appropriate temperatures and sterilizing the instruments. The autoclave, chemical vapor, and dry heat sterilizers are all appropriate tools for sterilization.

Sterilization of equipment is not, however, the only issue in dental office safety. The American Dental Association (ADA), the Centers for Disease Control (CDC), and the Occupational Safety and Health Administration (OSHA) have all issued guidelines for infection control in the dental office. It is up to you, however, to determine if the office in which you are being treated is following all the guidelines.

Once you have chosen a dentist and made your first visit, observe the instruments, the trays, the dental chair on which you are sitting, and the x-ray and other equipment. There is less chance of contamination when disposable instruments are used. Notice whether the tray on which the instruments are placed is covered by a disposable cover. If not, chances are the tray is either sprayed with a disinfectant or wiped, which may not thoroughly clean it of any blood and residue. If the instruments on the tray are not disposable, notice whether they are in a sterilized bag, or whether an assistant brought them out of a drawer. The sterilized bag is preferred.

The drill should either be disposable or come from a sterile bag. Burs used to drill the teeth, dispensers of cotton pellets, or any materials used on another patient should never be placed on the same tray with your instruments. Notice whether the assistant handles instruments with gloves, and whether the gloves are changed before a new patient's instruments are handled. The dentist must also wear gloves as well as a mask. He or she should not write on charts or answer the phone while wearing gloves. Handling an object may contaminate both the gloves as well as the object; it is another way of spreading disease.

While you are in the treatment room, notice if the chair you are sitting on has a headrest cover, and whether the dental light above the chair has disposable covers on the handles. In general, does the equipment and the room look clean? Any signs of shortcuts or lack of cleanliness are warnings.

In addition to observing the office for cleanliness, consider the dentist's use of safety devices during certain procedures. One such device is a "dental dam"—a square rubber sheet that exposes the tooth or teeth that are being treated. Most endodontists use it to prevent contamination of the pulp chamber. Some dentists use the dam when removing fillings from teeth to protect the throat from loose particles or filling materials. Because it is time-consuming to place, most dentists don't use it. Make sure a dental dam is used for root canal therapy, and consider suggesting that your dentist use it when filling your teeth.

Trust your judgement. Most dental office personnel feel somewhat intimidated when asked questions regarding sterilization techniques, even though they are routinely asked in this day and age. Therefore, it is important to observe closely the office and the personnel and make your decision, not strictly on how nice everyone is, but also on how professional and clean the office appears.

Remember, the risk of contracting AIDS or any communicable disease or infection can be minimized by proper sterilization and cleanliness. Furthermore, it is very important that any patient who has a communicable disease informs the health-care professional of his or her medical history. This will allow the staff to take appropriate precautions.

WHAT EXPENSES ARE INVOLVED IN VISITING THE DENTIST?

Although safety is of paramount importance when choosing a dentist, cost is also a genuine concern. Within a specific geographic region, most dentists charge essentially the same for the same procedure. Take all of the preceding factors into consideration when comparing costs. If you feel the fees are overly expensive, you should keep looking.

Holistic dentistry is an area that has become more popular in recent years. However, many so-called holistic dentists charge more than general dentists but don't do anything different. Some holistic dentists perform unnecessary tests while charging exorbitant fees.

If cost is a problem, consider being treated at a dental school (a list of these schools is provided beginning on page 203). Treatments are performed by third- and fourth-year dental students under the watchful eyes of their instructors. Here, you can receive excellent treatment for less than you would pay a dentist in private practice. Be aware, however, that each appointment takes about three hours. (Most dental instructors and professors have private practices at the school; however, they charge private-practice fees.) City clinics that provide emergency care for low fees are also available. Check with a local dental society for a list of such clinics. Some local hospitals also have clinics that charge low fees; for example, Santa Monica Hospital in California has a low-fee program offering full dental care for minors. Call your local hospitals and inquire about such services.

IN WHAT INSURANCE PLANS/ PAYMENT PROGRAMS DOES THE DENTIST PARTICIPATE?

There are three main types of dental insurance: the health maintenance organization (HMO), preferred provider insurance (PPI), and indemnity insurance. Because the programs are expensive, few employers offer dental benefits. Some dental insurance plans can be obtained on an individual basis.

If you are looking for a dental insurance plan for yourself, your family, and/or your business, check with your insurance agent or look in your local *Yellow Pages* under "Insurance." You can also call the American Dental Association's Department of Public Information and Education at 312–440–2593 to request a copy of *Selecting a Dental Benefits Plan.* (There is no charge for single copies.)

Before enrolling in any dental plan, be sure you understand how the program works, which procedures are covered, and what costs are involved. Each type of insurance has advantages and disadvantages of which you should be aware.

The HMO usually costs the insured less on a monthly basis. With an HMO, the insurance company contracts with dental or medical offices in various areas. The insured selects one of these offices and may seek services only at that location. To visit another location, the insured must contact the insurance company to make necessary arrangements. The contracted provider receives a set amount of money per insured person. Basic services such as exams, cleanings, and fillings are pro-

vided at no charge to the insured; however, more extensive treatments such as crowns and bridges have a set copayment that the insured must pay. The disadvantage of the HMO is that the copayments are usually low, and the provider often prefers not telling the patient about some needed treatments since he or she would lose money. If you require only preventive care and not extensive treatment, this is an adequate type of insurance.

With PPI, the insured also chooses doctors from a list, but the doctors under contract usually receive a certain prearranged percentage (usually 70 percent) of their usual and customary rate. Under this arrangement, you are more likely to receive the proper diagnoses and treatment for extensive problems, since the provider receives adequate compensation. The premiums for PPI are more than those for an HMO but less than those for indemnity insurance.

With indemnity insurance, you choose the doctor you will visit. Your insurance contract specifies the percentage of the doctor's usual and customary rate (UCR) that the insurance company will pay for each treatment. For example, 100 percent of the exams, cleanings, and x-rays might be covered; 80 percent of the fees for fillings; and 50 percent of the doctor's usual fee for crowns, dentures, and bridges. With this type of insurance, you have a maximum dollar amount you can spend on treatment per year, and you have a deductible. Indemnity insurance is more expensive, but the advantage is that you can choose any doctor you want, and you will receive all needed treatment.

Dentists who accept only indemnity insurance are more likely to offer payment plans. Some dentists will allow you to charge their services to a major credit card. If your bill is large, some dentists will be willing to work out a schedule of weekly or monthly payments until the bill is paid in full. If paying the bill is a concern for you, be sure to discuss payment options before beginning treatment.

Choosing a dentist is not simply a matter of walking into the office nearest you. You want safe, professional, caring treatment at a reasonable cost, and you can find it if you do your homework.

Part Two

Common Dental Disorders

Introduction

In Part One, you were introduced to the basics of dental health and to several natural approaches to dental care. In Part Two, the most common dental-related disorders are presented in alphabetical order. Each entry begins with a brief description and/or explanation of the condition, followed by information about the conventional treatments used to control the disorder. Nutritional supplements, homeopathic treatments, and herbal treatments appropriate to the disorder are then presented in easy-to-read chart form. In many cases, the charts refer you to Part Three, where you can find further information, such as directions for preparing various herbal remedies. Where appropriate, information about emergency treatment appears in the outside margin next to the entry. Each entry ends with recommendations for helping yourself, and, in some cases, references to pages on which you can find more information. Because each treatment category is not necessarily useful for every problem, some entries do not include all the treatments.

No one should care more for your health than you. Ask questions, and learn all that you can. The information in Part Two will enable you to take a more active role in your dental health.

In a number of cases, the descriptions of certain conditions may help you determine if you have a particular problem. If your symptoms match those given for a specific disorder, you can confirm your suspicions by visiting your dentist. Once a diagnosis has been confirmed, you can refer to the appropriate entry. Should you have any questions about the appropriateness of any suggested remedy, you may wish to speak to the proper professional health-care provider.

In other cases, your dentist may call a problem to your attention. In such cases, the appropriate entry can be referred to for suggested self-care options. Again, a professional health-care provider should be consulted if you have any questions about these options.

Abrasion

Abrasion refers to loss of tooth surface due to overzealous brushing, the clasp of a partial denture, braces, or from harsh, gritty toothpaste. Chewing on hard objects such as pencils, toothpicks, paperclips, and hairpins can also cause tooth abrasion. Carpenters who use their teeth to hold nails and garment workers who continually use their teeth to hold pins may cause notches to be abraded into the tooth enamel where the object was held. Those who polish stones, woods, and metals for a living and professional blasters who are exposed to dust and do not practice proper daily oral hygiene may expose themselves to tooth abrasion. When loss of tooth surface is not due to mechanical wear and occurs mostly near the gum line, it is referred to as erosion.

Abrasion and erosion may affect any part of a tooth. The affected area may appear worn away. If an area is slightly abraded or eroded, no change in color is noted; however, if wear has reached the dentin, the area will usually be a yellowish color. If the cause of the abrasion is not removed or halted, then damage will continue, ultimately leading to sensitivity and pain. Once the cause is removed, further damage is prevented. What's done is done, though, and the abraded area will remain damaged unless treated by a dentist.

CONVENTIONAL TREATMENT

Slightly abraded areas may be smoothed. Local fluoride applications or rinses may be recommended to temporarily relieve sensitivity. Low-abrasion toothpastes such as Sensodyne, Thermodent, and Grace contain ingredients to help reduce the sensitivity of abraded teeth. For long-lasting relief for an abraded area that is painful and has become extensively damaged, fillings and crowns will be recommended. Furthermore, it is important to determine the cause of the abrasion in order to eliminate the problem. Ill-fitting partials must be adjusted to prevent further wear. Improper use of a toothbrush or other hygiene aids should be corrected.

NUTRITIONAL SUPPLEMENTS

Supplement	Directions for Use	Comments
Calcium	Take 1500 mg daily.	Important part of healthy bones and teeth; helps relieve the tension associated with grinding and clenching of teeth.
Magnesium	Take 750 mg daily.	Works with calcium in bone; is involved in transmission of nerve impulses.
Thiamin (vitamin B$_1$)	Take 100 mg daily.	Involved in transmission of nerve impulses; may be helpful for reducing pain sensitivity.
Vitamin D	Take 10 mcg daily.	Important in absorption of calcium, which is necessary not only for strong teeth and bone, but also for proper functioning of the nervous system.

HOMEOPATHIC TREATMENT

When using tablets, dissolve them under your tongue. Do not eat or drink for fifteen minutes prior to or after taking medication. (See Part One, Homeopathy, for additional information.)

Preparation	Directions for Use	Comments
Belladonna 30X	Take 1 tablet 3 times a day or hourly for throbbing pain.	Helps reduce tooth pain and the grinding of teeth.
Chamomilla 30X	Take 2 tablets twice a day.	Helps reduce toothache and sensitivity to hot.
Plantago major 6X	Take 1 tablet 3 times a day as needed.	Helps reduce toothache caused by sensitivity to cold.

HERBAL TREATMENT

Herb	Directions for Use	Comments
Chamomile	Prepare as tea (see Part Three, Using Herbs, Tea Preparation). Drink 2–3 cups per day.	Induces relaxation.
Cloves	Add ¼ teaspoon of powder to a few drops of water. Prepare a salve (see Part Three, Using Herbs, Application Preparation). Apply to sensitive area 3 times a day.	Soothes tooth sensitivity.
Hops	Prepare as tea (see Part Three, Using Herbs, Tea Preparation). Drink 1 cup before bedtime.	Produces relaxation and sleep.

RECOMMENDATIONS

■ Avoid lemons, limes, and extremes of cold or hot foods or drinks if sensitivity exists.

■ Use low-abrasion toothpastes, such as Sensodyne, Grace, and Thermodent, which contain ingredients to help reduce tooth sensitivity.

Abscess

An abscess is a swelling filled with pus. There are three types of dental abscesses that resemble each other; it is their point of origin that differentiates them. A *gum or gingival abscess* is the result of injury to or infection of the surface of the gum tissue. If an infection moves deep into gum pockets, drainage of pus is blocked and a *periodontal abscess* results. A *periapical abscess* refers to a tooth in which the pulp is infected, usually secondary to tooth decay (see figure on following page).

A gum abscess is the result of irritation caused by toothpicks or other objects, from food being forced into the gums, or by aggressive brushing. If the trauma causes a break in the gum surface, bacteria invade the area, causing a local infection. Initially, the area appears red, smooth, and shiny. As the infection progresses, the area becomes pointed and pus is released.

A periodontal abscess involves the deeper structures surrounding the tooth. This kind of abscess develops when the gum pocket becomes blocked by plaque, tartar, and/or food. Because these foreign substances are not removed daily, harmful bacteria proliferate, resulting in a series of reactions. In response to the presence of these substances, the body's immune system sends particular cells to fight the foreign substances and the harmful bacteria contained in the plaque. Studies have shown that more than one type of harmful bacteria cause gum disease and the resulting abscess. Some types of bacteria found at various stages of gum disease, including abscesses, are *Bacteroides*, *Actinobacillus*, *Actinomyces*, *Capnocytophaga*, and *Treponema*. The resulting infections are caused by the reaction between the toxins of these bacteria and the immune cells present to destroy the bacteria.

A tooth-related or periapical abscess is usually a result of damage to the nerve of the tooth, and is present along with swelling, pain, reddening of the gums, and sensitivity to chewing and/or hot or cold. The tooth related to the abscess usually has a deep cavity or filling. Pus is caused by destruction of tissue by toxins and interruption of the blood supply. The center of the abscess absorbs fluid from surrounding tissue, causing the abscess to become larger. Fever, malaise (feeling tired, no energy), and swelling in the neck area may be present with the abscess. The infection may stay localized or spread. If an abscess is deep, a fistula (a tubelike passage from the abscess to the surface of the gums) forms where the fluids are released. However, if the fluids in the abscess are released into the surrounding tissues instead of being discharged on the surface, the infection spreads and is called cellulitis. Fever, chills, and lack of appetite increase as the infection worsens.

A condition called cementoma, in which excess bone forms around the root of a

FIRST AID

✚ If an abscess has a pimple-like swelling at the tip, rinsing with warm salt water will cause it to form a head, which will eventually release pus. Over-the-counter ointments may help relieve symptoms such as pain, and burning. Do not use over-the-counter steroid ointments since these may cause infections to spread.

✚ Aloe vera gel, *Belladonna* 30x, and *Silicea* 6x applied directly to abscessed area, and mouthwashes made of dandelion or a combination of echinacea, myrrh, and licorice may provide temporary relief.

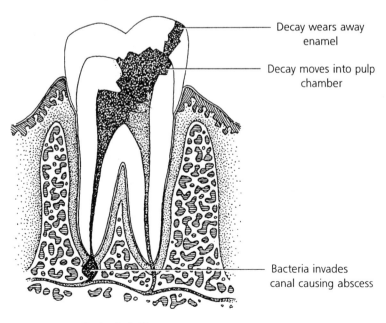

Decay wears away enamel

Decay moves into pulp chamber

Bacteria invades canal causing abscess

Periapical Abscess

tooth or teeth, looks like an abscess during its beginning stage, but it is not. Cementoma, often caused by trauma, is usually seen on lower front teeth. No treatment is required.

An abscess may have a sudden appearance (acute) or it may have been present for a long period of time (chronic) without any signs or symptoms. In the acute stage, the gums around the abscess become enlarged, red, tender, and painful. The tooth may be loose and sensitive to chewing. Pressing on the area where the gums and teeth meet may release pus. A dull pain that throbs and radiates may be present. Periodontal abscess may produce a feeling of sickness, fever, and swelling in the lymph glands in the neck. If the infection has been present for a long time (chronic), there may be no symptoms. Treating the acute abscess is more successful than treating the chronic, which has caused more extensive damage over time.

CONVENTIONAL TREATMENT

It is important to determine which type of abscess is present so that the appropriate treatment may be rendered. In all three types of abscess, the pus must be drained. Antibiotics may be prescribed if systemic symptoms such as fever and swelling in the lymph glands are present. (Mouth infections often affect the lymph glands in the neck region.) Deep cleaning will be suggested for gum pocket (periodontal) abscesses. If too much bone has been lost and the tooth is too loose, it may have to be pulled. In the case of a periapical abscess, root canal therapy (see Endodontic Techniques, Root Canal Therapy, in Part Three) or tooth extraction is indicated.

NUTRITIONAL SUPPLEMENTS

Supplement	Directions for Use	Comments
Garlic	Take 500 mg 3 times daily.	Acts as an antibacterial.
Vitamin B_6	Take 100 mg daily.	Increases oxygen to cells through manufacture of hemoglobin.
Vitamin B_{12}	Take 100 mg daily.	Important to normal cell growth and function.
Vitamin C	Take 2000 mg daily.	Enhances healing.
Zinc	Take 30 mg daily.	Enhances healing.

HOMEOPATHIC TREATMENT

When using tablets, dissolve them under your tongue. When using liquids, place the drops directly on your tongue. (Because of their alcohol base, liquids should not be used by children or recovering alcoholics.) Do not eat or drink for fifteen minutes prior to or after taking medication. (See Part One, Homeopathy, for further information.)

Preparation	Directions for Use	Comments
Belladonna 30X	Take 10 drops or 1 tablet every ½ to 1 hour, depending on the severity of the pain.	Indicated for throbbing pain and fever.

Calcarea fluorica 6X	Take 4 drops or 2 tablets daily.	Indicated for chronic abscess; may take time before it clears infection.
Silicea 6X	Take 2 drops or 1 tablet 3 times a day.	Indicated if teeth are sensitive to cold after pus is discharged.
Hepar sulphuris 6X	Take 2 drops or 4 tablets each hour.	Promotes discharge of pus.

HERBAL TREATMENT

Herb	Directions for Use	Comments
Chamomile	Prepare as tea (see Part Three, Using Herbs, Tea Preparation). Drink 3–4 cups daily. If face is swollen from infection, prepare poultice (see Part Three, Using Herbs, Application Preparation) and apply to cheek outside the affected area one or more times daily until abscess is drained.	Promotes drainage of pus.
Echinacea	Prepare as a mouthwash (see Part Three, Using Herbs, Mouthwash Preparation). Rinse with a warm solution every 2 hours.	Promotes healing.

RECOMMENDATIONS

■ As diabetics are prone to the spread of infections, they should notify their dentist and physician at the first sign of an abscess.

■ Avoid alcohol and sugar, but drink large amounts of water, grape juice, and grapefruit juice, and maintain a low-fat diet.

■ Decrease iron intake. As reported in the *American Journal of Nutrition* in 1982, excessive iron supplementation can release toxins that hasten bacterial growth.

■ *See also* Plaque in Part Two.

Acute Necrotizing Ulcerative Gingivitis

See Gum Disease.

AIDS-Related Dental Problems

SOURCES OF HELP

For information on AIDS or for help in dealing with the condition, contact:

AIDS Action Committee
131 Clarendon Street
Boston, MA
617–437–6200

AIDS Hot Line
800–342–2437

American Foundation for AIDS Research
733 Third Avenue
12th Floor
New York, NY 10017
212–682–7440

National Association of People With AIDS
1413 K Street, NW
7th Floor
Washington, DC 20005
202–898–0414

Project Inform
347 Dolores Street #301
Dept. P
San Francisco, CA 94110
800–822–7422

AIDS (acquired immune deficiency syndrome) causes the body to lose its ability to defend itself against infections or other illnesses. This immune deficiency ultimately leads to death. The virus that causes AIDS is HIV (human immunodeficiency virus), and is transmitted in a variety of ways. Since contaminated blood is a main source of infection, those receiving blood transfusions, intravenous drug users, and health-care providers are at high risk for contamination.

Dental problems are often the first signs of AIDS. Sore, bleeding gums and herpes sores appear in the mouth. Fever may be present. As the syndrome progresses, severe gum disease develops. There is no apparent cause, and the gum disease is difficult to control. Herpes, fungal infections, and candida (yeast) infections spread in the mouth, and the sides of the tongue develop a hairy appearance. The glands under the jaw become swollen, and purplish blotches appear on the roof of the mouth. Because of these symptoms, AIDS patients often visit the dentist before consulting with any other health-care provider.

Due to the nature of dental treatment, many fear that AIDS may be transmitted during treatment. Precautionary safety measures including proper sterilization of dental equipment is critical in minimizing the risk of AIDS transmission (see Choosing a Dentist in Part One).

CONVENTIONAL TREATMENT

Care must be taken to follow proper hygiene methods at home on a daily basis. If brushing teeth is difficult because the surrounding gum tissues are too tender, use a cotton-tipped applicator to clean the teeth and gums. A thorough cleaning by a dentist or hygienist is important; however, as AIDS progresses, the gums become extremely tender and a professional cleaning may become too painful.

NUTRITIONAL SUPPLEMENTS

Supplement	Directions for Use	Comments
Garlic	Take 500 mg 6 times daily.	Has antibiotic properties; helps strengthen immune system.
Vitamin B complex	Take 100 mg daily.	Improves various complex activities involved in normal cell growth and function.
Vitamin C	Take 6000 mg daily.	Repairs connective tissue; has antioxidant properties; helps stop and prevent bleeding of gums.
Zinc	Take 60 mg daily.	Enhances healing of sores.

HOMEOPATHIC TREATMENT

When using tablets, dissolve them under your tongue. When using liquids, place the drops directly on your tongue. (Because of their alcohol base, liquids should not be used by children or recovering alcoholics.) Do not eat or drink for fifteen minutes prior to or after taking medication. (See Part One, Homeopathy, for additional information.)

Preparation	Directions for Use	Comments
Apis mellifica 30X	Take 3 tablets or 6 drops 3 times daily.	Indicated for swollen gums, sore tongue, and sore throat.
Capsicum 6X	Take 1 tablet or 4 drops 3 times daily.	Helps to heal herpes sores and reduce inflammation.

HERBAL TREATMENT

Herb	Directions for Use	Comments
Aloe vera	Place gel on a cotton-tipped swab (see Part Three, Using Herbs, Application Preparation), and apply to gums sparingly at bedtime. Do not eat or drink for at least 1 hour after applying the gel.	Has soothing, astringent properties.
Anise and sage	Prepare together as tea (see Part Three, Using Herbs, Tea Preparation) and use as a mouthwash as needed.	Has soothing effect on painful, inflamed gums.

RECOMMENDATIONS

■ Strengthening the immune system and ensuring proper oral hygiene are extremely important in minimizing the progress of AIDS and its related diseases.

■ Since the gum tissues become very tender, avoid the use of hard-bristled or electric toothbrushes, alcohol mouthwashes, and harsh toothpastes. Grace Toothpaste is a mild paste that contains vitamin C, baking soda, and aloe vera, and is available at most stores where toothpaste is sold.

■ *See also* Gum Disease; Oral Herpes Infections; Yeast Infection in Part Two.

Anesthesia-Related Problems

See Anesthesia in Part Three.

Anorexia-Related Tooth Disorders

See Eating Disorders and Tooth Problems.

Antibiotic-Related Problems

Antibiotics are used to fight bacterial infections. They may be taken in pill or liquid form, or used as a mouthwash and then swallowed. Antibiotics are also given by injection. Produced by bacteria, molds, and fungi, antibiotics have the power to destroy or inhibit the multiplication of other types of organisms, especially bacteria. Some antibiotics are effective against fungi and a few viruses as well.

Penicillin, erythromycin, and tetracycline are the most commonly prescribed antibiotics in dentistry. Usually taken for gum infections and abscesses, antibiotics are also commonly prescribed after extractions of infected teeth and during root canal therapy. If certain medical conditions such as a heart murmur are present, antibiotics are prescribed before any treatment to prevent infection.

Once an antibiotic is ingested, it may be toxic to intestinal bacteria. Desirable ("friendly") bacteria as well as undesirable ones will, therefore, be poisoned and destroyed. This leaves the intestinal walls unprotected against irritating or unabsorbed foods, causing inflammation of the tissues. Similarly, if an antibiotic is taken for a long period of time, the particular strain of bacteria it is meant to destroy may eventually become resistant. As a result, mutant strains of bacteria are produced. Another side effect to long-term intake of a particular antibiotic is that by destroying bacteria, it produces an imbalance in the microorganism population. For example, intestinal candida, which is a yeast organism, proliferates with long-term antibiotic use because much of the bacterial population is destroyed. (See Yeast Infection in Part Two.)

Antibiotics may produce an assortment of gastrointestinal complaints and a variety of allergic reactions that range in seriousness from a mild rash to shock and even death. In addition, most antibiotics interfere with the estrogen in birth control pills, rendering the pills inactive. Blood cholesterol levels are raised by some antibiotics, since the bacteria that help rid the body of cholesterol are destroyed by the drug.

Since its discovery in 1941, penicillin has been the antibiotic used for the majority of dental infections. The occurrence of side effects depends on how well an individual tolerates the drug. A person allergic to penicillin will usually experience a reaction within half an hour of taking the drug. In some allergic reactions, the muscles in the throat become constricted, causing breathing difficulty. In more serious reactions, the capillaries dilate, causing shock, which, if not treated immediately, can lead to death.

Other side effects of penicillin use reveal themselves from two hours to three or more days after taking the medication. These include fever, mental changes, edema (abnormal accumulation of fluid in tissues), abnormal heartbeat, inflammation of the kidneys and renal failure, swollen tongue, many types of skin rashes, and inflammation of any or all parts of the mouth. Because penicillin crosses the placental barrier and is excreted in mother's milk, its use should be avoided during pregnancy and lactation.

The antibiotic of choice for individuals allergic to penicillin is erythromycin, which was first used in 1952. Although food reduces erythromycin absorption, it may be necessary to take this drug with meals because of its adverse effect on the gastrointestinal tract. Erythromycin is distributed to most body tissues and excreted via the liver in the bile, and in urine and feces. Side effects associated with erythromycin include gastrointestinal irritation, abdominal cramps, nausea, vomiting, and diarrhea. All the side effects disappear when the drug is discontinued. Individuals taking digoxin, warfarin, or carbamazepine, and those taking theophylline for asthma or bronchitis, may experience adverse reactions to erythromycin and should, therefore, avoid taking it.

Discovered in 1948, tetracycline is a broad-spectrum antibiotic that affects a wide range of microorganisms. It concentrates in the liver and is excreted into the intestines via the bile. This drug should not be taken by pregnant or lactating women or by children between the ages of two months and eight years because of its side effects. Tetracycline is secreted in the saliva and the milk of lactating women, and is stored in the unerupted teeth of nursing babies. When the teeth erupt, they have permanent stains (see Teeth, Stained in Part Two), which darken with age and exposure to light. A decreased growth rate in bones has also been demonstrated in infants and fetuses who have ingested and/or been exposed to tetracycline.

Although tetracycline is prescribed for severe gum disease, it should be taken with caution because of its many adverse side effects. Some of these side effects include lightheadedness, dizziness, and vertigo. People taking this drug should not drive or perform any hazardous jobs. In addition, tetracycline reacts negatively with antacids, iron, oral contraceptives, barbiturates, and warfarin. With long-term ingestion of tetracycline, the targeted organisms may become resistant to the medication. Because the resistant strain of bacteria cannot be destroyed by any antibiotic, the condition is called a "superinfection."

There are other antibiotics prescribed in dentistry, but like the above antibiotics, they should be taken with caution and only when absolutely necessary.

✍ **TAKE NOTE**

Organisms may become resistant to an antibiotic after long or repeated treatment. It is, therefore, very important to use antibiotics only when necessary, in the correct dosage, and for the prescribed time period.

NUTRITIONAL SUPPLEMENTS

Supplement	Directions for Use	Comments
Vitamin B complex	Take 100 mg daily.	Helps maintain normal cell growth and function.
Garlic	Take 250 mg 3 times a day.	Acts as a natural antibiotic.

HOMEOPATHIC TREATMENT

Dissolve the tablets under your tongue. Do not eat or drink for fifteen minutes prior to or after taking medication. (See Part One, Homeopathy, for additional information.)

Preparation	Directions for Use	Comments
Acidum nitricum 30X	Take 1 tablet 2 times a day.	Helps control diarrhea caused by antibiotics.
Borax 30X	Take 1 tablet 3 times a day.	Good treatment for thrush (candida) of the mouth and intestines.
Nux vomica 30X	Take 1 tablet hourly.	Helps relieve gastric disturbances.
Pyrogenium 30X	Take 1 tablet daily.	Useful when there is risk of infection.
Sulphur 30X	Take 1 tablet daily.	Helps to alleviate rashes on skin.

HERBAL TREATMENT

Herb	Directions for Use	Comments
Glucomannan	Take 1 gm, ½ hour before meals 3 times daily.	Helps eliminate toxic substances produced during digestion.
Goldenseal	Take 1 tablespoon of powder 3 times a day. May be sprinkled on food.	Soothes irritated lining of stomach, intestines, and spleen.

RECOMMENDATIONS

■ Remember, infections are less likely to occur and antibiotics will not be needed if you keep your immune system strong and healthy, practice proper nutrition, and exercise regularly.

■ Most of the ill effects of antibiotics are due to the imbalance they cause in the normal bacteria of the body. To maintain the proper balance, eat eight ounces or more of yogurt daily (goat's milk yogurt if you have an allergy to cow's milk), acidophilus milk, or kefir (cultured milk products in which *Lactobacillus acidophilus* bacteria are growing).

■ Decrease or avoid consumption of meat or other animal products that cause fermentation in the intestines.

■ Even if you have filled out a medical history form, review with your dentist the medications you are taking. If the dentist gives you a prescription, talk to the pharmacist about the drugs you are taking. Most pharmacists are well-informed about the latest research and information on drug interactions.

■ Remember, antibiotics block the effects of oral contraceptives.

■ Alcohol interacts negatively with antibiotics and must be avoided.

■ Pregnant and lactating women should avoid antibiotics unless they are absolutely necessary.

■ Dated antibiotics or medicine in bottles with no expiration dates should be discarded immediately.

■ Do not share antibiotics or other prescription medications with other people.

Anxiety

See Pain and Anxiety in Part Two; and Stress and Anxiety Management in Part Three.

Aphthous Ulcers

See Canker Sores.

Bad Breath (Halitosis)

Bad breath may be caused by gum disease, tooth decay, dehydration, digestive disturbances due to poor diet, alcohol, smoking, and some systemic diseases. Sulfur gases released by bacteria under the gums, ill-fitting crowns or dentures, and old, broken, or worn-out fillings may also cause bad breath. Early morning halitosis is primarily due to dehydration. During sleep, metabolism slows down, decreasing the flow of saliva. This allows acids and other debris to putrefy in the mouth, which is why it is so important to brush and floss thoroughly at bedtime. Dehydration is also the cause of bad breath in mouth-breathers. When the tissues in the mouth are overexposed to air, the mouth becomes dry, increasing the possibility of bad breath. Drinking adequate amounts of water helps keep the tissues healthy.

Diseases such as cancer cause a foul mouth odor. Those who suffer from renal disease will exhibit bad breath due to the discharge of urea in the mouth. Acetone breath is associated with diabetes and sinus infections. Constipation and colon congestion also cause bad breath. One way to test if you have bad breath is to cover your mouth and nose with your hand, exhale, and smell your breath.

CONVENTIONAL TREATMENT

Your dentist or hygienist may recommend commercial mouthwashes to eliminate bad breath; however, alcohol rinses should be avoided. If other symptoms are present along with the bad breath, your dentist may recommend that you be evaluated for systemic disease.

NUTRITIONAL SUPPLEMENTS

Supplement	Directions for Use	Comments
Chlorophyll	Take tablets or capsules as directed on package.	Eliminates bad breath.

Selenium	Take 100 mcg daily.	Increases oxygen utilization.
Vitamin B$_1$	Take 50 mg daily.	Neutralizes toxins in tissues.
Vitamin E	Take 600 IU daily.	Has antioxidant properties; works well with selenium; enhances oxygenation of blood.

HOMEOPATHIC TREATMENT

Dissolve the tablets under your tongue. Do not eat or drink for fifteen minutes prior to or after taking medication. (See Part One, Homeopathy, for additional information.)

Preparation	Directions for Use	Comments
Arnica 30X	Take 1 tablet daily.	Indicated for bad breath after tooth extraction.
Kali phosphoricum 12X	Take 1 tablet 3 times daily.	Indicated when diarrhea accompanies bad breath, and for morning dry mouth.
Mercurius solubilis 30X	Take 1 tablet 3 times daily.	Indicated when there is excessive saliva or gum disease.
Nux vomica 30X	Take 2 tablets daily.	Indicated for heavily coated tongue.
Pyrogenium 30X	Take 1 tablet daily.	Indicated for dry throat and dry, red, cracked tongue.

HERBAL TREATMENT

Herb	Directions for Use	Comments
Alfalfa	Prepare as tea (see Part Three, Using Herbs, Tea Preparation). Drink 2–3 cups daily, or take tablets or capsules as directed on package.	Purifies blood, clears constipation, removes toxins from tissues.
Cloves	Chew the seeds.	Helps eliminate bad breath.
Fennel	Chew the seeds.	Helps eliminate bad breath.
Kelp	Take tablets or capsules as directed on package.	Contains approximately 30 trace minerals; removes waste, regulates metabolism, and detoxifies the intestines.
Parsley	Take tablets or capsules as directed on package.	Eliminates bad breath.
Thyme	Prepare as tea (see Part Three, Using Herbs, Tea Preparation). Drink 2–3 cups daily.	Balances gastric disturbances.

RECOMMENDATIONS

■ If you are unable to brush after every meal, eat mouth-cleansing fruits and vegetables, such as apples, carrots, parsley, and celery.

■ Eat yogurt, kefir, or acidophilus daily to improve digestion.

■ Once or twice a day, cleanse the internal system with an 8-ounce drink of warm water mixed with one tablespoon of apple cider vinegar and one teaspoon of honey. For further prevention of halitosis, drink at least eight 8-ounce glasses of water per day to prevent dehydration. You can add lemon or lime juice to the water to further reduce mouth odor.

■ Decayed teeth and gum disease must be treated, and proper hygiene employed daily in order to decrease the risk of bad breath that originates in the mouth.

■ When brushing your teeth, also be sure to brush your tongue. Bacteria accumulates on the tongue and results in bad breath.

Bell's Palsy

See Facial Paralysis.

Bleeding Gums

See Gum Disease.

Bottle Mouth Syndrome

Infants who drink from bottles containing sugared drinks, juices, formula, or even unsweetened milk are soaking their teeth with sugars that can predispose the mouth to infections and cavities. This practice is especially harmful if babies are allowed to sleep with bottles left in their mouths. The resulting condition, called bottle mouth or nursing bottle syndrome, is characterized by numerous cavities, first in the upper front teeth, and then in the upper and lower back teeth. Nursing bottles should never be used as a pacifier or an aid to sleep. Water in the bottle is not harmful, but if your older child demands something else, provide it in a glass with or without a straw and follow with water in the bottle. Your baby should be weaned to a bottle or a cup no later than age one.

NUTRITIONAL SUPPLEMENTS

Supplement	Directions for Use	Comments
Vitamin C	Infants up to 1 year should have 35 mg daily; children age 1 through 10 should have 50 mg.	Important for healthy gums and teeth.

HOMEOPATHIC TREATMENT

Because of their alcohol base, liquid homeopathic preparations should not be given to children. Tablets, which have a sweet milk sugar base and can be dissolved in the mouth, are excellent for children. For infants, dissolve the tablet in water and give with an eyedropper. (See Part One, Homeopathy, for additional information.)

Preparation	Directions for Use	Comments
Kreosotum 30X	Give 1 tablet 2 times per week.	Indicated to help children relax and for anxiety control.

HERBAL TREATMENT

Herb	Directions for Use	Comments
Peppermint	Prepare mild tea (see Part Three, Using Herbs, Tea Preparation); add a dash of cinnamon for flavor. Cool and give to child.	Excellent for decay prevention.

RECOMMENDATIONS

■ Do not let children fall asleep with bottles of milk or juice in their mouths.

■ It is best to have the cavities associated with bottle mouth filled as soon as possible. If the cavities are left untreated, infection and pain may result.

Braces-Related Problems

Problems involving the growth and development of the teeth and the jaw are corrected by the use of braces and other orthotic appliances designed by an orthodontist. It is estimated that 50 percent of all children as well as many adults require orthodontic treatment.

Orthotic appliances affect speech and appearance while they are worn. Several problems that can have lasting effects on the teeth, gums, head, and neck area may present themselves during treatment. Severe gum swelling, stains on the teeth, and cavities may occur. Wires and braces present hard-to-clean surfaces, which easily accumulate food and plaque, and can eventually cause gum problems and cavities. If any bleeding or swelling is noticed while brushing, there is the potential for gum problems. Proper daily hygiene is essential, and it is very important to get regular dental checkups every six months during orthodontic treatment.

Braces or appliances are adjusted monthly to bring about the desired results, which may take from a few months to a few years. Following the adjustment of braces, some pressure and possibly pain is felt immediately or up to three days later. If the pain is severe, either the wires are too tight or teeth are being forced to move too rapidly, which may result in bone damage. Let the orthodontist know if the pain is severe so that he or she can adjust the tension of the wires, allowing the movement of the teeth to be accomplished at a slower, more comfortable rate.

Head gear or appliances worn in the mouth to affect the structure of bone may cause head, neck, and jaw problems (e.g. temporomandibular joint syndrome) years after treatment has stopped. During the initial consultation, the orthodontist will give you details about your treatment. If he or she tells you that treatment will affect bone structure, you should also consider seeing an osteopath (one who practices manipulative techniques for correcting certain bodily abnormalities). Osteopathic physicians are very familiar with the skeleto-muscular system and will make the appropriate preventive adjustments to your head, neck, and jaw during treatment. Look in your local *Yellow Pages* under "Physicians" for a listing of osteopathic physicians, or for osteopathic universities that you can contact for referrals. Call these physicians to see whether they routinely make cranial adjustments during orthodontic treatments or if they work with orthodontists during treatment. Chiropractors may also be consulted for similar adjustments.

Once the treatment is completed, further growth and development or natural forces may cause the teeth to assume their old position. This may be avoided if retainers are worn. If you notice any change in the position of your teeth after the completion of orthodontic treatment, consult with your orthodontist.

CONVENTIONAL TREATMENT

Your orthodontist will recommend regular dental checkups and professional cleanings to help keep braces-related problems in check. Proper home hygiene is also essential. Your orthodontist may recommend pain medication when wires are adjusted; however, the pain usually subsides within three to five days, and, if necessary, a nonprescription pain reliever such as Tylenol or Advil can be just as effective.

NUTRITIONAL SUPPLEMENTS

Supplement	Directions for Use	Comments
Calcium	Adults take 1500 mg daily; children, 360–800 mg daily.	An important component of healthy bones and teeth.
Coenzyme Q-10	Adults take 60 mg daily; children, 15 mg daily.	Improves circulation and, therefore, increases oxygen levels in tissues.
Magnesium	Adults take 750 mg daily; children, 50–350 mg daily.	Aids calcium assimilation.
Vitamin C	Adults take 2000 mg daily; children, 45 mg daily.	Helps to maintain healthy gums.

HOMEOPATHIC TREATMENT

Dissolve the tablets under your tongue. Do not eat or drink for fifteen minutes prior to or after taking medication. (See Part One, Homeopathy, for additional information.)

FIRST AID

✚ If a broken orthodontic appliance is bent or sharp, try to gently bend the wire back, but be careful, as the wire may break. If the appliance is irritating to the gums, place a piece of wax or chewed sugarless gum on the broken area until you see your orthodontist.

✚ Drink comfrey or marigold tea to relieve pain.

✚ If gums are inflamed, rinse with a mouthwash of chamomile, goldenseal, marigold, or peppermint, or drink anise tea.

Preparation	Directions for Use	Comments
Aconite 30X	Take 1 tablet hourly as needed.	Helps relieve neck pain after adjustments.
Amica 30X	On day of adjustment, take 1 tablet 1 hour prior to the appointment, 1 tablet 6 hours after the appointment, and 1 tablet at bedtime.	Helps relieve sore, painful muscles caused by appliance adjustment.
Ruta 6X	Take 2 tablets twice daily.	Helps relieve pain after adjustment of braces.

HERBAL TREATMENT

Herb	Directions for Use	Comments
Aloe vera	Place gel on a cotton-tipped swab (see Part Three, Using Herbs, Application Preparation). Apply directly to gums. Do not eat or drink for at least 1 hour after applying the gel.	Helps soothe irritated gums.
Comfrey	Prepare as tea (see Part Three, Using Herbs, Tea Preparation). Drink 2–3 cups daily. Dried powder or leaves may be sprinkled on food.	Helps relieve pain right after adjustment of braces.
Eucalyptus oil	Place on a cotton-tipped swab and rub on gums.	Helps to heal irritated gums.
Kelp	Take 400-mg tablets or capsules three times a day.	Contains minerals essential to healthy bones and teeth.
Marigold	Prepare as tea (see Part Three, Using Herbs, Tea Preparation). Drink 2–3 cups daily. Dried powder or leaves may be sprinkled on food.	Helps relieve pain right after adjustment of braces.

RECOMMENDATIONS

■ Children should take a multivitamin/mineral supplement daily.

■ While being treated orthodontically, have dental checkups and professional cleanings every three to six months.

■ Obtain some wax from your orthodontist for emergency use. If irritation occurs on the gums near a wire and the dentist is not available, place a small amount of wax under the wire to prevent further damage until the wire can be adjusted. Most local drug stores sell containers of wax in the oral hygiene section for this use. If none is available, you may improvise and place a piece of chewed sugarless gum or a piece of clean rubber band under the wire.

■ Rinsing your mouth with a mixture of eight ounces of warm water, one teaspoon of salt water, and one teaspoon of baking soda will help relieve irritated gums.

■ To relieve a jaw made sore by orthodontic treatment, or a sore neck if head gear is worn, apply moist heat (see Using Herbs, Application Preparation in Part Three). Acupressure may also be helpful (see Acupressure in Part Three).

■ Keep all appointments for adjustments to your braces, and follow all instructions.

■ Store removable appliances in a specific place where they won't get lost or damaged.

■ When involved in active sports, remove head gear or removable appliances.

■ Avoid hard or sticky foods. They will be difficult to clean off your braces or appliances and may even damage or break the appliance itself. Never chew gum, ice, or hard fruits or vegetables such as apples or carrots, unless you cut them into small pieces.

■ *See also* Orthodontic Techniques in Part Three.

Bridge-Related Problems

A bridge is a prosthetic device that replaces a few—usually up to three or four—missing teeth. There are three types of bridges: a fixed bridge, a bonded bridge, and a removable bridge (see Prosthodontic Techniques, Bridges, in Part Three). All bridges require that the teeth on either side of the missing teeth have strong bone and healthy gums.

Many different metals are used in bridges. Some people may be sensitive to one or more of the metals used. For instance, the gum tissue in contact with the metal may become irritated and start to recede. You can avoid problems related to sensitivity by testing for allergies before having the bridge made. If possible, obtain a sample of the metal that will be used, and leave the metal in contact with your skin for forty-eight hours. If no changes are noted on the skin, this particular metal is safe to use.

Imbalanced bite is a problem associated with fixed bridges. An imbalanced bite can be created at any stage, beginning with the trimming of the tooth up to the point when the laboratory fabricates the bridge. However, whatever the cause, imbalanced bite can usually be corrected before the bridge is cemented. The dentist uses a corrective tape on the bridge to determine where the imbalance is, then corrects the problem with a drill. If the imbalance is not corrected and the bridge is cemented, trauma from excessive force will create pain. The pain will be felt mostly when you are chewing. If the bridge contains porcelain, it may fracture.

Chewing gum or eating foods such as taffy may loosen a fixed bridge. Usually, bridges can be recemented. If the bridge does not fit tightly against the teeth, cavities can begin to form in the teeth on which the bridge is placed. Cavities can also form here if proper hygiene is not practiced.

A bonded bridge consists of one or more artificial teeth attached to metal wings that are bonded to the natural teeth. The problems experienced with this type of bridge are similar to those experienced with a fixed bridge. A bonded bridge is more likely to become loose, since the wings are bonded to only one surface of the natural teeth. A bonded bridge—appropriate for replacing lower front teeth, which are not used for heavy chewing—should be bonded to teeth that are cavity-free.

The removable bridge consists of an artificial tooth or teeth attached to a metal framework that rests on the adjacent teeth by means of clasps. This type of bridge

FIRST AID

✦ Over-the-counter products sold in drug stores can be used to temporarily cement broken bridges and crowns. If you wear a bridge or a crown, keep one of these products in your medicine cabinet.

✦ To soothe irritated gums, rinse with chamomile or goldenseal mouthwash, or apply aloe vera gel directly to sore area.

is the least expensive, but it is also the least desirable. It is the most uncomfortable and the most likely to become loose.

When you get any type of bridge, initially your gums may be sensitive and tender for a short period of time. If teeth have been missing for a long time, bone and gums may have resorbed. An artificial tooth placed here may look fake because there will be a space between it and the gum.

For further information on bridges, see Prosthodontic Techniques in Part Three.

CONVENTIONAL TREATMENT

To ease tender gums when you first get a bridge, your dentist will probably recommend that you rinse with warm salt water for a week. Pain medication may also be prescribed if pain is anticipated. If teeth appear fake due to resorption, a gum specialist may graft tissue to build up the gums and cover the space.

NUTRITIONAL SUPPLEMENTS

Supplement	Directions for Use	Comments
Vitamin C	Take 500 mg daily.	Enhances tissue repair.
Zinc	Take 80 mg daily.	Promotes healing.

HOMEOPATHIC TREATMENT

Dissolve the tablets under your tongue. Do not eat or drink for fifteen minutes prior to or after taking medication. (See Part One, Homeopathy, for additional information.)

Preparation	Directions for Use	Comments
Hypericum 30X	Take 1 tablet 3 times a day for a week.	Use after major dental work to aid in recovery of damaged nerves.
Mercurius solubilis 30X	Take 1 tablet 3 times a day.	Use one day before the appointment and for one week after treatment to counteract any harmful effects of mercury in amalgams that may need to be removed or placed during treatment.

HERBAL TREATMENT

Herb	Directions for Use	Comments
Aloe vera	Place gel on a cotton-tipped swab (see Part Three, Using Herbs, Application Preparation). Apply directly to gums. Do not eat or drink for at least 1 hour after applying the gel.	Promotes healing of irritated, sore gums.

Chamomile	Prepare tea (see Part Three, Using Herbs, Tea Preparation); allow to cool and use as a mouthwash 2–3 times a day.	Very soothing for irritated gums.
Goldenseal	Prepare tea (see Part Three, Using Herbs, Tea Preparation); allow to cool and use as a mouthwash 2–3 times a day.	Very soothing for irritated gums.

RECOMMENDATIONS

■ Discuss thoroughly with your dentist the different types of bridges and their advantages and disadvantages for your particular situation. Know the type of metal that will be used in the appliance.

■ It may take one week or longer to get used to a new bridge. If, however, pain is experienced while chewing, your bite may not be correct on the bridge, which may cause trauma to the teeth and their supporting structures. Immediately inform the dentist of the situation, and have the bridge adjusted as soon as possible.

■ From the first appointment in having the bridge made, to two weeks after it has been completed, try not to chew hard foods. Having been drilled, the teeth have been traumatized and require time to recuperate. Chew soft foods after first receiving the bridge, and gradually introduce harder foods until the area feels completely normal.

■ *See also* Implants; Prosthodontic Techniques in Part Three.

Broken, Cracked, or Chipped Teeth

Natural and artificial teeth can become chipped, cracked, or broken. The usual cause of a tooth's becoming chipped is trauma. A person bites on something hard, bumps the tooth on some object, or puts excessive force on a tooth by grinding or clenching the teeth, and a chip occurs. There is often no pain associated with a chip; sometimes, the person does not even know how it happened. Depending on the size of the chip, it can be smoothed or cosmetically corrected. If a filling or an artificial tooth becomes chipped, it is replaced.

Cracks or fractures in teeth can be caused by the same events that cause a chip; however, they involve more damage. For example, if the force is strong enough, the crack will affect the root surface. Cracks are not always visible, even on x-rays. The symptoms involve pain on chewing, at times accompanied by sensitivity to cold and hot. The pain may initially be weak and occasional, eventually becoming more pronounced and frequent.

There are many circumstances that can cause a tooth to break. A molar with an excessively large filling may not have enough tooth surface to withstand the forces of chewing, and may break when a hard food is chewed. New cavities may form

FIRST AID

✚ If you are in pain from a broken, cracked, or chipped tooth, take an over-the-counter pain medication such as Tylenol or Advil. If possible, keep any part of the tooth that has broken off, especially if it is a gold or porcelain filling, which may be recemented.

✚ If a hole is apparent in the tooth and is causing pain, saturate a cotton ball with oil of cayenne, clove, peppermint, or summer savory and place it in the hole. You can also drink chamomile tea or soak a washcloth in warm comfrey tea and use it as a compress.

under old fillings, weakening the tooth; without warning, the filling and parts of the tooth may break. If a root-canaled tooth is not protected by a crown, breakage is common due to the brittleness of the dead tooth. Broken teeth should be treated immediately.

CONVENTIONAL TREATMENT

Cracked and broken teeth should be repaired as soon as possible to prevent further damage. If the pain from a crack or fracture is severe, root canal therapy or tooth extraction may be necessary. If the crack affects the enamel and dentin of the tooth, a crown is the best choice of treatment.

If there is no pain involved with a chipped tooth and the chip is small, it's up to you to decide if, when, and how the tooth should be repaired. There are many options available for repairing chipped teeth including veneers, crowns, fillings, and simple smoothings of the chipped areas. Ask your dentist to explain these options. (See Cosmetic Dentistry; Prosthodontic Techniques in Part Three.)

NUTRITIONAL SUPPLEMENTS

Supplement	Directions for Use	Comments
Calcium	Take 1500 mg daily.	Important component of healthy bones and teeth.
Magnesium	Take 750 mg daily.	Works with calcium for healthy bones and teeth.
Multivitamin and multimineral	Give to children as directed by pediatrician.	Promotes healing and anxiety.
Vitamin C	Take 1000 mg daily.	Has anti-inflammatory properties.

HOMEOPATHIC TREATMENT

Dissolve the tablets under your tongue. Do not eat or drink for fifteen minutes prior to or after taking medication. (See Part One, Homeopathy, for additional information.)

Preparation	Directions for Use	Comments
Ammonium carbonica 6X	Take 1 tablet hourly.	Relieves severe tooth pain that accompanies chewing.
Chamomilla 30X	Take 1 tablet hourly.	Relieves tooth pain that worsens when exposed to heat.
Hypericum 30X	Take 1 tablet 3 times a day.	Take after dental treatment to reduce pain and to prevent permanent or long-lasting nerve damage.

HERBAL TREATMENT

Herb	Directions for Use	Comments
Aloe vera	Place gel on a cotton-tipped swab (see Part Three, Using Herbs, Application Preparation). Apply directly to gums at bedtime.	Promotes healing.
Chamomile	Prepare as tea (see Part Three, Using Herbs, Tea Preparation). Drink 2–3 cups per day.	Has a soothing effect on a toothache and promotes relaxation and sleep.
Clove oil	Place on a cotton-tipped swab and rub on the affected tooth.	Helps relieve pain.
Hops	Prepare as tea (see Part Three, Using Herbs, Tea Preparation). Drink 2–3 cups per day.	Has a soothing effect on a toothache and promotes relaxation and sleep.
Marjoram	Prepare as tea (see Part Three, Using Herbs, Tea Preparation). Drink 2–3 cups per day.	Has a soothing effect on a toothache and promotes relaxation and sleep.

RECOMMENDATIONS

■ Have cracked or broken teeth repaired as soon as possible.

■ Do not chew hard foods with a newly cracked or broken tooth.

■ Avoid very hot or very cold foods or drinks.

■ If a huge hole is exposed in a tooth and you cannot get to a dentist immediately, place a cotton ball moistened with clove oil in the hole and seek treatment as soon as possible.

■ If your temporary crown comes off and the dentist is not available, purchase a temporary crown cement from your local drug store. Follow the instructions on the package. Temporarily cementing the crown in place will help prevent further problems from developing. (If the temporary crown is not recemented, the tooth may move or crack further.)

■ Try not to chew hard foods on a new crown for a few days until the crown feels normal.

■ *See also* Trauma to Children's Teeth in Part Two; and Cosmetic Dentistry; Prosthodontic Techniques in Part Three.

Bruxism

Bruxism or tooth grinding usually occurs during sleep. This unconscious habit, which is generally believed to be caused by stress, can result in loose and worn teeth, gum recession, and destruction of the supportive bones of the teeth. After a prolonged history of bruxing, patients may run the risk of problems involving the jaw joint, such as temporomandibular joint syndrome (TMJ). Treatment for bruxism is similar to that recommended for TMJ. See TMJ in Part Two.

Bulimia-Related Tooth Disorders

See Eating Disorders and Tooth Problems.

Cancer, Oral

See Oral Cancer.

Candidiasis

See Yeast Infection.

Canker Sores (Aphthous Ulcers)

DID YOU KNOW . . .
Canker sores are very similar in appearance to cold sores, which are caused by the contagious herpes virus. Herpes or cold sores are likely to be found on the hard part of the gums and the outer part of the lips. They tend to recur in the same spot. Canker sores are found on the loose part of the gums and the insides of cheeks and lips.

Canker sores are small, white swellings that change into ulcers (open sores sometimes accompanied by pus) surrounded by an area of redness. Appearing suddenly, their most painful phase lasts three to six days. Canker sores are more common in women and usually begin to appear by the age of twenty. The attacks decrease with age.

Although the cause of canker sores has never been proven, predisposing factors in some people may include deficiencies in iron, folic acid, or vitamin B_{12}. Genetic tendency, trauma, cigarette smoking, allergies to certain foods, stress, and immunologic factors (e.g. HIV infection) have also been implicated as possible causes.

CONVENTIONAL TREATMENT

Your dentist may recommend mouth rinses such as Dexamethasone elixer, topical preparations such as Kenalog in Orabase (ointment), and mild pain relievers to help alleviate canker sore pain. Frequently, corticosteroids are prescribed by the dentist. Antibiotics and experimental vaccines have not been proved beneficial. A blood analysis will indicate if deficiencies of vitamin B_{12}, iron, or folic acid are present.

NUTRITIONAL SUPPLEMENTS

Supplement	Directions for Use	Comments
Folic acid	Take 400 mcg daily.	Important in development of red blood cells; deficiency may cause canker sores.
Garlic	Take two 250-mg capsules 3 times daily.	Acts as a natural antibiotic.
Iron	Take 18 mg daily.	Helps relieve fatigue, a possible cause of canker sores; deficiency is also a possible cause of the sores.
Vitamin B_{12}	Take 200 mcg daily.	Deficiency may cause canker sores.
Vitamin C + bioflavonoids	Take 3000 mg daily.	Promotes healing.
Vitamin E	Frequently apply oil to sores, especially when they first appear.	Promotes rapid healing.
Zinc	Take 30 mg daily.	Promotes healing.

HOMEOPATHIC TREATMENT

Dissolve the tablets under your tongue. Do not eat or drink for fifteen minutes prior to or after taking medication. (See Part One, Homeopathy, for additional information.)

Preparation	Directions for Use	Comments
Borax 30X	Take 1 tablet 3 times daily as needed.	Helps relieve pain and reduce inflammation from canker sores.
Antimonium crudum 6X	Take 1 tablet 3 times daily as needed.	Helps heal canker sores.
Natrum muriaticum 30X	Take 1 tablet 3 times daily as needed.	Helps relieve burning and itching from canker sores.

FIRST AID

✛ Mouth sores will heal by themselves; however, over-the-counter ointments and aloe vera gel may help relieve symptoms such as pain and burning. Do not use over-the-counter steroid ointments since these may cause infections to spread.

✛ When canker sores appear on lips and cheeks, use *Natrum phosphoricum* 6X; when they appear between gums and lips, use *Rhamnus californica* tincture. (Topical or internal homeopathic preparations may be used.)

HERBAL TREATMENT

Herb	Directions for Use	Comments
Burdock	Take 500-mg tablet daily as needed.	Helps purify blood.
Goldenseal	Take 400-mg tablet daily as needed.	Acts as an anti-inflammatory.
Red clover	Take 400-mg tablet daily as needed.	Acts as an anti-inflammatory and helps purify blood.

RECOMMENDATIONS

■ During periods of active flare-up, avoid alcoholic beverages, chocolate, chewing gum, lozenges, coffee, and strawberries. Hard, crusty foods, irritating foods such as potato chips and nuts, and spicy, hot foods such as pizza may exacerbate the sores.

■ Plain yogurt (cow or goat milk), kefir, and acidophilus should be consumed daily. Eat plenty of fruits and vegetables, and drink grape and carrot juices, which are particularly safe and gentle on the ulcerated tissue.

Cavities (Dental Caries)

A cavity or tooth decay is a bacterial disease that affects all the structures or layers of the tooth. Tooth decay is very much influenced by lifestyle—specifically one's family and social environment. In Western society, cavities are the most common human disorder.

When the environment in the mouth becomes too acidic, calcium and phosphate ions are lost from the enamel crystals that constitute the surface layer of the tooth. If the acidity level remains, bacteria, especially *Streptococcus mutans*, and other organisms produce toxins from ingested sugars. These toxins form a sticky mass that allows food debris and bacteria (plaque) to stick to the tooth surface. The plaque acts as a direct application of acid to the teeth, further demineralizing the enamel and leading to cavities. The chances for cavity formation increase with increasing consumption of carbohydrates. Similarly, the more refined the carbohydrates in your diet, the greater the chances for cavity formation.

If the loss of minerals continues, the tooth surface begins to disintegrate and the cavity becomes deeper. If the loss of minerals ceases and new minerals are deposited, then the cavity stops growing and somewhat reverses. However, this reversal occurs only at the surface layer or enamel of the tooth. Once the bacteria have reached the dentin, or inner layer, the cavity usually continues to grow.

Cavities are more prone to develop in pits on top of the back teeth, in between the teeth, and near the gum area where the bristles of a toothbrush cannot reach. Soft root surfaces, exposed when gums have receded, develop cavities that spread to other surfaces of the tooth.

The rate at which a cavity progresses depends on the bacteria involved and the body's resistance to disease. This is true for disease in any part of the body, but resistance to dental disease also depends on heredity, diet, hygiene, fluoride content of teeth, and general dental health.

The first sign of a cavity is a white spot. Depending on the factors listed above, it will stay like this or progress to a brown color.

CONVENTIONAL TREATMENT

The dentist uses a tool called an explorer (see Figure 3.6 on page 174) and x-rays to determine the extent and depth of the cavity. Usually, if the spot is in the tooth's enamel, no treatment is needed. If the spot has extended into dentin, which will be evident on the x-ray, treatment is required. Treatment depends on the size and depth of the cavity. A small cavity can be filled. Filling materials can be amalgam, composite resins, porcelain, or gold. (For detailed information on treatment for cavities, see Filling a Cavity in Part Three.)

NUTRITIONAL SUPPLEMENTS

Supplement	Directions for Use	Comments
Calcium	Take 1500 mg daily.	An important component of strong, healthy teeth.
Magnesium	Take 750 mg daily.	Works along with calcium to maintain healthy teeth.
Zinc	Take 30 mg daily.	Influences growth, immune function, and healing.

HOMEOPATHIC TREATMENT

When using tablets, dissolve them under your tongue. When using liquid, place the drops directly on your tongue. (Because of their alcohol base, liquid homeopathic preparations should not be given to children. Tablets, which have a sweet milk sugar base and can be dissolved in the mouth, are excellent for children.) Do not eat or drink for fifteen minutes prior to or after taking medication. (See Part One, Homeopathy, for additional information.)

Preparation	Directions for Use	Comments
Arnica 30X	Take 1 tablet every 15 minutes as needed.	Helps relieve toothache pain that is worse at night.
Chamomilla 30X	Take 1 tablet hourly as needed.	Indicated for toothache that worsens in response to heat.
Hypericum 30X	Take 1 tablet 3 times daily.	Take immediately after treatment to promote nerve healing and prevent pain.
Mercurius solubilis 30X	Take 1 tablet 3 times daily.	To remove any residue of mercury in mouth, begin taking the preparation on the day of the treatment, and continue for 4 days.
Plantago major (tincture)	Take 5 drops hourly as needed.	Use when toothache is more sensitive to cold.

FIRST AID

✚ Over-the-counter products containing lidocaine or benzocaine, such as Anbesol, Orajel, and Campho-Phenique, can be used topically to provide temporary relief for toothache. Over-the-counter pain relievers such as Tylenol are also helpful. Do not rub aspirin or other analgesics on the gums. These contain strong acids and may burn the gum tissues. A small piece of cotton saturated with clove oil and placed on the tooth will give temporary relief. Avoid sweets and hot and cold foods.

✚ Over-the-counter products can be used to plug a cavity until you see the dentist. Or you can make your own temporary filling by mixing 1 tablespoon of powdered goldenseal with 1/2 teaspoon of warm water until a smooth paste is formed; add 1 drop of clove oil and mix till smooth. Place the mixture in the hole with a rounded toothpick or the wooden end of a cotton-tipped swab.

✚ Use a chamomile poultice (see Part Three, Using Herbs, Application Preparation) or drink hot hops tea (see Part Three, Using Herbs, Application Preparation) for relief of pain. Take Arnica 30X for a toothache that is worse at night. Use Plantago major tincture for a toothache that is sensitive to the touch and worsens in the presence of cold.

HERBAL TREATMENT

Herb	Directions for Use	Comments
Chamomile	Prepare as a tea (see Part Three, Using Herbs, Tea Preparation). Drink 2–3 cups daily or use as a mouthwash.	Tea promotes relaxation; mouthwash eases sore teeth and gums after a cavity is filled.
Clove oil	Place on cotton-tipped swab and rub on tooth.	Helps relieve tooth pain.

RECOMMENDATIONS

■ Take no more than 2000 mg of vitamin C on the day of treatment. Excessive amounts of the vitamin decrease the effectiveness of oral anesthetics.

■ For best results, it is recommended to use the same filling material (if the material has a metal component) for all of the cavities in your mouth. Some studies show that a galvanic reaction or battery effect may result when different metals are placed in the mouth. Currents are generated from a metal when it contacts saliva; this effect is compounded when different metals, such as those from gold fillings and amalgam fillings, are present in the same mouth. Some experience this effect as a shock when a fork touches a particular filling. However, nonmetallic filling materials, such as porcelain and composite resins, can be used in conjunction with metal fillings without causing a galvanic reaction.

■ Pregnant and breastfeeding women should have cavities filled only in an emergency. Dental anesthetics cross the placental barrier, and x-rays, stress, and trauma experienced during a dental visit may affect the unborn baby. It is generally safest to have teeth filled during the fourth through seventh months of pregnancy. The most hazardous times are the first and last trimesters, when the baby is at the most crucial stages of its development.

■ *See also* Filling a Cavity in Part Three.

Cellulitis

See Abscess.

Cementoma

See Cysts and Tumors.

Cheek-Biting

See Lip- and Cheek-Biting.

Chipped Tooth

See Broken, Cracked, or Chipped Teeth.

Cleft Palate and Lip

A cleft forms when two bones don't join (fuse). Cleft lips and/or palates occur in approximately one of every seven hundred live births in the United States. A cleft palate forms when the bones in the palate do not join. As a result, there is a hole or crack in the middle of the roof of the mouth, as seen in the top margin figure. The cleft lip shown in the middle figure consists of one or more splits in the upper lip caused by the failure of the upper jaw and nasal area to close in the embryo. Cleft lip and cleft palate may occur in the same individual, as seen in the bottom figure.

Clefts have a tendency to run in families, but the actual cause has not been determined. Hormonal imbalances, nutritional deficiencies, toxic substances in drugs, and certain anesthetics (e.g., nitrous oxide) when used during pregnancy have been implicated as possible causes.

Clefts create many problems for newborn infants; some of which may not be reparable until the child becomes older. Surgical repair is usually begun when the child is one or two years of age. If damage to the bony palate is extensive, surgery may be delayed until the child is between five and seven to prevent structural problems. Eating, breathing, speech, and psychological problems are some of the difficulties confronted by the child with a cleft lip or palate. Correction of these conditions calls for teamwork involving a plastic surgeon, maxillofacial surgeon, otolaryngologist (ear, throat, larynx, and pharynx specialist), general dentist, orthodontist, and oral surgeon.

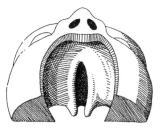

Cleft Palate

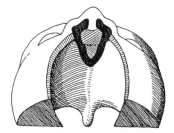

Cleft Lip

CONVENTIONAL TREATMENT

Infants who have clefts will require multiple corrective surgeries over an extended period of time. The plastic and maxillofacial surgeons perform corrective surgery on the face, while the general dentist, oral surgeon, otolaryngologist, and orthodontist make appliances to correct any defects. Surgical closure of the cleft lip is accomplished as soon as the infant is able to withstand the general anesthesia and

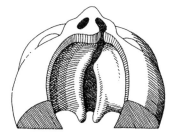

Cleft Palate and Lip

surgery. This is usually within three to four months after birth. Surgery for closure of the palate is delayed until initial speech development, when the upper jaw has reached normal growth. If after surgery, the upper jaw has somewhat collapsed so that the teeth do not meet properly, orthodontic treatment will correct the condition. In some cases, surgery is not possible or it may not totally close the hole. In this case, a denturelike appliance is made to cover the hole and allow normal eating.

The health-care team will provide guidance and encouragement during the difficult time from birth to corrective treatment. With the advances in surgical techniques and orthotic appliances, the prognosis for cleft lips and palates is excellent. As the child gets older, little sign of the cleft will remain.

NUTRITIONAL SUPPLEMENTS

Supplement	Directions for Use	Comments
Vitamin B complex	Give 25 mg daily.	Helps enhance the immune system.
Vitamin C	Give 200 mg daily.	Helps promote healing after corrective surgery.

HOMEOPATHIC TREATMENT

Because of their alcohol base, liquid homeopathic preparations should not be given to children. Tablets, which have a sweet milk sugar base and can be dissolved in the mouth, are excellent for children. For infants, dissolve the tablet in water and give to the child with an eyedropper. (See Part One, Homeopathy, for additional information.)

Preparation	Directions for Use	Comments
Chamomilla 30X	Give 3 drops hourly.	Helps calm an irritable and restless infant.
Rheum 30X	Give 1 drop hourly.	Helps calm an irritable and restless infant.

HERBAL TREATMENT

Herb	Directions for Use	Comments
Alfalfa	Prepare as tea (see Part Three, Using Herbs, Tea Preparation). Add 1 teaspoon of honey if the child is older than 1 year. Allow to cool and give the baby 4 ounces in a bottle daily.	Acts as an antioxidant and improves healing. Rich in minerals.
Catnip	Prepare as tea (see Part Three, Using Herbs, Tea Preparation). Allow to cool and give the baby 4 ounces in a bottle daily.	Excellent for calming irritability.

RECOMMENDATIONS

■ Infants with cleft palate and/or lip require special care and handling. Be sure to hold the infant upright when feeding and use a specially made nipple that has an extended tip and large holes. Hold the nipple in contact with the baby's cheeks or soft palate so the liquid does not get into the breathing passages.

■ If sucking is difficult, use a rubber bottle, squeezing it gently as the baby feeds.

■ If surgery has recently been performed on the lip, it is preferable to use a medicine dropper for feeding instead of a bottle, which requires sucking. Breast-feeding is not recommended.

Cracked Lips

See Lips, Cracked.

Cracked Tooth

See Broken, Cracked, or Chipped Teeth.

Crown, Lost

An artificial crown is made to replace tooth enamel that is extensively damaged. Crowns may be made of metal, gold, or porcelain. Although crowns can withstand greater chewing forces than bonded teeth, they do sometimes fall out.

CONVENTIONAL TREATMENT

If the crown is intact, the dentist can clean the tooth and recement the crown. If the crown is broken, a new one is necessary.

RECOMMENDATIONS

■ If you have a crown or bridge, be sure to keep an over-the-counter dental cement in your medicine cabinet. This product can be used to temporarily cement a crown or bridge in place until you can see your dentist.

■ See also First Aid; Prosthodontic Techniques, Crowns in Part Three.

Cysts and Tumors

A cyst is a hollow sac or pouch that contains fluid, semifluid, or solid material and may form in soft tissue or bone. It usually results from developmental abnormalities, obstruction of ducts, or infection. Eruption cysts are caused by erupting teeth and are benign. These cysts will rupture as the teeth erupt and require no treatment. Cysts in the mouth may also be the result of trauma. A variety of cysts affect the mouth; some are associated with the teeth and others with the jawbone. All are painless, but speaking or eating may irritate them, causing some discomfort. Cysts in the jaws make the bones more likely to fracture. They may also cause teeth to become so loose that they eventually have to be pulled. Most cysts are benign; however, on rare occasions a cyst may undergo a malignant transformation.

A tumor is an abnormal growth of soft tissue or bone and may be benign or malignant. There are many types of tumors and, with a few exceptions, their causes are not known.

One type of nonmalignant tumor in the mouth is an oral tori. This growth of bone may occur in the lower or upper jaw, which includes the palate, in a variety of sizes and patterns. No treatment is necessary unless the tumor becomes irritated or interferes with the wearing of dentures, in which case, it must be surgically removed. Oral tori are fairly common and follow a hereditary pattern.

The tooth-related tumor known as a cementoma is an accumulation of the bonelike connective tissue that covers the roots of the tooth or teeth. This tissue proliferates abnormally. When x-rayed in its initial stage, a cementoma may look similar to an abscess. Because of this similarity, root canal work may be performed unnecessarily. As a cementoma develops, fibrous tissue replaces bone in the area of the tumor, and the problem becomes easy to diagnose. A cementoma is often the result of an injury, and usually occurs in groups of teeth, usually the lower front teeth near the end (apex) of the roots. They are seen more often in women, have no symptoms, and require no treatment.

During the first trimester of pregnancy, benign growths called pregnancy tumors sometimes appear in the soft supporting tissue between adjacent teeth. They are characterized by a reddish mass that grows rapidly. The overlying skin is thin and tends to crumble. The area bleeds easily and does not blanch when pressure is applied. These tumors may last throughout the pregnancy and may or may not subside after the birth of the child. Pregnancy tumors may be removed surgically or through the application of electrical current.

CONVENTIONAL TREATMENT

Treatment for cysts varies depending on the type. Most are surgically removed while others are drained. One type that usually does not require surgery is the eruption cyst. Tumors, on the other hand, are never drained, but are either left alone or surgically removed. A biopsy is usually performed to determine the type and status of a tumor. In this procedure, a small sample of the tumor tissue is removed, mounted on a glass slide, and examined microscopically. If the tumor is found to be malignant, chemotherapy or radiation therapy may be recommended.

NUTRITIONAL SUPPLEMENTS

Supplement	Directions for Use	Comments
Beta-carotene	Take 25,000 IU daily.	May prevent cancer; important in maintaining healthy mucous membrane (inner lining of the mouth).
Coenzyme Q-10	Take 60 mg daily.	Improves circulation and increases the level of oxygen in tissues.
Vitamin B complex	Take 100 mg daily.	Important in normal growth and development of cells.
Vitamin C	Take 2000 mg daily.	Acts as an antioxidant and promotes healing.
Zinc	Take 30 mg daily.	Important in the healing of sores.

HOMEOPATHIC TREATMENT

Dissolve the tablets under your tongue. Do not eat or drink for fifteen minutes prior to or after taking medication. (See Part One, Homeopathy, for additional information.)

Preparation	Directions for Use	Comments
Calcarea fluorica 6X	Take 1 tablet 2 times daily.	Indicated for tumors and cysts of the jaw.
Hekla lava 6X	Take 1 tablet daily.	Indicated for tumors and cysts of the jaw.
Viscum album 30X	Dosage is determined by a physician and administered by injection.	Indicated for malignant tumors; stimulates immune response.

HERBAL TREATMENT

Herb	Directions for Use	Comments
Alfalfa	Prepare as tea (see Part Three, Using Herbs, Tea Preparation). Drink 2–3 cups daily or take tablets or capsules as directed on the package.	High in minerals and an effective antioxidant.
Elderberry	Prepare as mouthwash (see Part Three, Mouthwash Preparation). Rinse with ½ cup daily.	Promotes healing after surgery; good source of vitamin C.

RECOMMENDATIONS

■ If you notice any type of swelling in your mouth, it is important to seek professional diagnosis.

■ A balanced diet with fresh fruits and raw or steamed vegetables and grains is advisable. You should also drink at least eight 8-ounce glasses of water daily.

■ If you have a tori, be careful when eating hot or crusty foods—pizza, potato chips, French bread—as they may cause irritation.

■ Pay attention to any changes in the shape or size of any tumor. Some tumors, like the tori, may never change. However, if you notice a change in any tumor, see a dentist immediately.

■ *See also* Oral Cancer in Part Two.

Dental Caries

See Cavities.

Denture-Related Problems

FIRST AID

✚ Products such as Quick Fix and Plate-Weld are available at drug stores and may be used for temporary repair of the denture or of the teeth that have broken off it.

✚ To relieve irritated or inflamed gums, rinse with a mouthwash made of anise, goldenseal, marigold, myrrh, peppermint, or sage. Rub eucalyptus oil or evening primrose oil on the affected gums.

✚ To relieve ulcers caused by dentures, rinse with marigold or rockrose mouthwash.

✚ Use *Antimonium crudum* 6X, *Arum triphyllum* 30X, or *Natrum muriaticum* 30X to relieve cracks at the corners of the mouth.

When dental decay or gum disease affects a majority of the teeth, the dentist may remove all the teeth and replace them with artificial teeth or dentures. Troublesome dentures can be downright embarrassing. Their appearance can keep you from smiling, and they may sometimes be loose enough to fall out at the most inappropriate times. Ill-fitting dentures can also cause difficulty in speaking and/or eating. However, in this modern day of dentistry, there is help. Dentures can be very natural looking; also, they can be comfortable enough to resolve speech and eating problems.

New dentures always present some challenges, and it may take time to get used to them. One of the most common problems associated with new dentures, although it can occur with an old denture also, is sores. Sore gums are usually caused by new dentures that have been left in for too long, and from chewing on hard foods before your tissues have had a chance to adjust. If your gums do get sore, take the dentures out and frequently rinse your mouth with warm salt water. Wait a few days until the sores have healed, and then try the dentures again. If your mouth still feels sore, see your dentist. After adjustments are made, gradually increase the number of hours you wear the dentures. Although this may seem time-consuming, you will adjust to your dentures more easily this way and have fewer sores and less irritation to your gums.

If an immediate denture is placed in your mouth after tooth extraction, you will be told to leave it in for the next twenty-four hours. Follow your dentist's instruction. (For more information on the fitting and fabrication of immediate dentures, see Prosthodontic Techniques in Part Three.) In the privacy of your home, practice talking and reading out loud. Look in the mirror while you make different facial expressions. This will help you get used to your new dentures.

You may find that your dentures simply do not fit well due to improper construction. Ill-fitting dentures, which may also result from smoking, stress, and poor nutrition, can damage the gums and bones. If ill-fitting dentures have been worn for a very long time, excess flaps of tissue will begin to form on the ridge where the denture sits. If the borders of the dentures are too long in either direction they may cause mouth ulcers, which will heal eventually, leaving flanges—flabby or excessive gum tissue—in their place. If the flanges get in the way of the dentures, the extra tissue may have to be surgically removed, and new dentures will have to be made.

Dentures may cause cracks in the skin at the corners of the mouth. If dentures do not have the overbite (the vertical extension of the upper teeth over the lower teeth) best suited for your jaw alignment, the skin at the corners of your mouth may become creased. This, in turn, causes saliva to accumulate in those corners, causing macerations or cracks. These irritated, burning cuts can also be due to deficiencies of iron, vitamin B or C, or folic acid. You need to determine whether the dentures or nutritional deficiencies are causing the cracks, so that the proper corrections can be made.

Overbite is also directly related to a balanced jaw relationship. Improper vertical alignment of the teeth (improper overbite) may, therefore, cause problems with your jaw joint. You may experience radiating pain to the temples while chewing, and may find that you cannot pronounce certain letters such as "s" properly. If the dentures are not placed properly, cheek and tongue biting may occur.

If redness under the dentures is accompanied by a burning sensation, you should suspect an allergic reaction. Some people are allergic to dental adhesives or cleansers, and even to materials in the dentures themselves. Sometimes, the allergy occurs because denture cleansers are not rinsed off thoroughly after use. Residue from the cleansers can irritate the gums and cause ulcers. Bacteria can then enter the tissue through the ulcers and cause more serious problems. Trial and error will determine the source of the allergy. Eliminate the cleansers, adhesives, and other materials one at a time, and wait for the reaction before eliminating the next item. If no change occurs, leave the dentures out and see what happens. The materials used in the dentures themselves may be the cause. In such cases new dentures made of different materials may be necessary.

If the area under the dentures becomes bright red but is painless, an endocrine imbalance (e.g., diabetes and adrenal insufficiency) or a candida infection may be the cause. The gum condition may be initiated by ill-fitting dentures and exacerbated by candida (see Yeast Infection, Oral, in Part Two). Leaving the dentures out, correcting the fit, and treating the candida will cure this condition.

Ill-fitting dentures can also cause gagging if the dentures are extended back too far in the roof of the mouth. Dentures with broken teeth and teeth with rough edges can traumatize the tongue and the gum tissues that come in contact with them.

Sometimes redness under the dentures is accompanied by small bumps that give the gums a raspberry appearance. This condition is caused by long-term irritation and the moving of rough denture surfaces over the gums. Removing the dentures and correcting the cause of the irritation usually clears the condition.

CONVENTIONAL TREATMENT

With most types of problems related to ill-fitting dentures, the dentist makes adjustments on the dentures and recommends that you leave the dentures out until the gums have healed. Adjustments are accomplished by smoothing rough edges or surfaces with a drill or by shortening long borders of the denture base. If too much adjustment is needed for the denture to fit properly, a new lining for the base of the dentures (a reline) is needed. The dentist may prepare the reline in his or her office or send the dentures to a laboratory. If the overbite is determined to be incorrect, the teeth may have to be reset on the dentures.

81

For cuts at the corners of the mouth, ointments such as Nystatin, Bacimycin, Mycolog, or Chlortetracycline may be prescribed. For candida infections, Nystatin lozenges, Ketoconazole tablets, or Clotrimazole troches (lozenges) are commonly prescribed. The dentist may also recommend improving denture hygiene by cleaning and storing dentures overnight in prescription solutions such as 0.2 percent chlorhexidine.

NUTRITIONAL SUPPLEMENTS

Supplement	Directions for Use	Comments
Calcium	Take 1500 mg daily.	Helps ensure health of jawbone upon which denture base rests.
Folic acid	Take 400 mcg daily.	Deficiency causes cracks in the corners of the mouth.
Garlic	Take 6 tablets daily of 250 mg each.	Acts as a natural antibiotic.
Kelp	Take 3 tablets daily of 500 mg each.	Has a balanced mineral content.
Magnesium	Take 750 mg daily.	Works with calcium in maintaining healthy bones.
Vitamin B_{12}	Take 100 mg daily.	Increases oxygen to tissues of the gums.
Vitamin C	Take 1500 mg daily.	Important for healing sore gums and maintaining healthy gums.

HOMEOPATHIC TREATMENT

Dissolve the tablets under your tongue. Do not eat or drink for fifteen minutes prior to or after taking medication. (See Part One, Homeopathy, for additional information.)

Preparation	Directions for Use	Comments
Arnica 30X	Take 1 tablet 3 times daily.	Take for relief of sore gums.
Arum triphyllum 30X	Take 1 tablet 3 times daily.	Indicated when corners of mouth are sore and cracked.
Kali muriaticum 6X	Take 1 tablet hourly.	Take when candida is present along with sore gums.

HERBAL TREATMENT

Herb	Directions for Use	Comments
Aloe vera	Place gel on cotton-tipped swab (see Part Three, Using Herbs, Application Preparation). Apply directly to gums. Do not eat for at least 1 hour after applying the gel.	Helps soothe and heal inflamed gums.

Anise	Prepare as mouthwash (see Part Three, Using Herbs, Mouthwash Preparation). Rinse with ½ cup, 2–3 times daily.	Excellent for relief of inflamed, tender gums.
Eucalyptus oil	Place on a cotton-tipped swab and rub on gums.	Helps heal gum sores.
Evening primrose oil	Place on a cotton-tipped swab and rub on gums.	Helps heal gum sores.
Goldenseal	Prepare as mouthwash (see Part Three, Using Herbs, Mouthwash Preparation). Rinse with ½ cup, 2–3 times daily.	Excellent for relief of inflamed, tender gums.
Marigold	Prepare as a mouthwash (see Part Three, Using Herbs, Mouthwash Preparation). Rinse with ½ cup, 2–3 times daily.	Excellent for relief of inflamed, tender gums and mouth ulcers.
Myrrh	Prepare as mouthwash (see Part Three, Using Herbs, Mouthwash Preparation). Rinse with ½ cup, 2–3 times daily.	Excellent for relief of inflamed, tender gums.
Peppermint	Prepare as a mouthwash (see Part Three, Using Herbs, Mouthwash Preparation). Rinse with ½ cup, 2–3 times daily.	Excellent for relief of inflamed, tender gums.
Rockrose	Prepare as a mouthwash (see Part Three, Using Herbs, Mouthwash Preparation). Rinse with ½ cup, 2–3 times daily.	Excellent for relief of inflamed, tender gums and mouth ulcers.
Sage	Prepare as a mouthwash (see Part Three, Using Herbs, Mouthwash Preparation). Rinse with ½ cup, 2–3 times daily.	Mild antiseptic.

RECOMMENDATIONS

■ Take your dentures out after meals and scrub them thoroughly. A hard toothbrush and baking soda toothpaste are safer than the harsh, irritating chemicals found in some commercial denture cleansers.

■ Leave your dentures out at night to promote circulation and rest for the tissues in your mouth. Scrub the dentures and soak them overnight in a solution of baking soda and water (one tablespoon of baking soda in enough water to just cover the dentures).

■ The procedure for making dentures usually requires three to four visits to the dentist. If it takes only one appointment, shortcuts were taken. For information on the fitting and fabrication of dentures, see Prosthodontic Techniques in Part Three.

■ If wearing the dentures makes your mouth sore, make an appointment with the dentist for an adjustment. However, as stated earlier, sores are less likely to occur if you get used to the dentures slowly.

Dry Mouth (Xerostomia)

Unfortunately, dry mouth (xerostomia) due to insufficient saliva, is a common problem. It can occur rapidly when a person experiences sudden anxiety, or it can be present all the time due to other causes. Menopause causes persistent dry mouth, as do pipe, cigar, and heavy cigarette smoking. This condition usually accompanies illnesses such as diabetes, blood disorders such as leukemia and pernicious anemia, Sjorgren's syndrome (a disease of the salivary glands), and immunosuppressed diseases such as Hodgkin's and AIDS. Radiation therapy involving the head and neck area, and some medications including tranquilizers, antidepressants, antihistamines, amphetamines, and hypotensives as listed in the table on page 85 also cause dry mouth. Dry mouth will be present until the causes are removed.

Mouth-breathing is a major cause of dry mouth, which, in turn, causes gum swelling and inflammation, especially around the front teeth. Mouth-breathing is caused by an inability to close the mouth due to an imbalance in the bite, or to blockage of nasal passages because of a deviated septum or enlarged adenoids.

Frequent side effects of a constantly dry mouth include a burning sensation on the tongue, a metallic taste, cracks in the corners of the mouth, numerous cavities, gum disease, and mouth sores. When dry mouth is present, the soft tissues of the oral cavity are more prone to infection. Because saliva has a buffering effect (reduces acidity), gum disease and cavities are usually worsened or caused by dry mouth. Bad breath (halitosis) is often present with dry mouth, due to the absence of the antiseptic, protective effect of saliva. The sense of taste may also be altered or diminished, and swallowing may become more difficult. Full dentures may not fit as well, since saliva enhances the ability of the dentures to adhere to the tissues. Not only will the denture not fit properly, but, as a direct result of dry mouth, it may irritate the gums.

CONVENTIONAL TREATMENT

Removing the cause of the dry mouth is the only effective long-term treatment. Temporary relief from dry mouth can be obtained by using mouth moisturizers such as Xerolube or Oralube as a saliva substitute. Using Biotene brand toothpaste, chewing sugarless gum, and rinsing with mouthwashes that are specially formulated to help dry mouth may also bring temporary relief. Fluoride applications and rinses are often prescribed to help minimize cavity development.

NUTRITIONAL SUPPLEMENTS

Supplement	Directions for Use	Comments
Coenzyme Q-10	Take 60 mg daily.	Improves circulation and increases oxygen to cells.
Vitamin B complex	Take 100 mg daily.	Important in development of healthy cells.
Vitamin C	Take 2000 mg daily.	Promotes and maintains healthy gum tissue.

Medications That Cause Dry Mouth

The following categories of prescription and over-the-counter drugs contain listings of pharmaceuticals that may cause dry mouth.

Analgesics
(used for pain relief)

Acetaminophen (Tylenol)	Aspirin Darvon	Demerol

Antianginals
(used for angina pectoris)

Calan	Cardizem	Procardia
Cardilate	Nitroglycerin	

Antiarrhythmics
(used for control of irregular heartbeat)

Calan	Procan SR	Xylocaine
Cardioquin	Pronestyl	
Isoptin	Quinaglute	
Norpace	Quinora	

Anticonvulsants
(used for prevention of epileptic seizures and treatment of stroke)

Dilantin	Zarontin
Tegretol	

Antidepressants
(used for treatment of depression)

Asendin	Loxitane	Sinequan
Desyrel	Ludiomil	Tofranil
Elavil	Norpramin	
Limbitrol	Pertofrane	

Antiemetics
(used for treatment of nausea, dizziness, vomiting)

Bonine	Reglan
Inapsine	Tigan
Marinol	Vontrol

Antihistamines
(used to help reduce and eliminate symptoms of allergy and inflammation)

Actidil	Contac	Phenergan
Actifed	Dimetane	Seldane
Antivert	Dristan	Teldrin
Atarax	Myridil	Temaril
Bonine	Optimine	Vistaril

Antihypertensives
(used for treatment of high blood pressure)

Aldomet	Lopressor	Vasotec
Apresoline	Minipress	Visken
Capoten	Normodyne	Wytensin
Catapres	Serpasil	
Corgard	Tenormin	
Inderal	Trandate	

Decongestants
(used to relieve stuffed nose and sinuses)

Afrin	Otriven
Neo-Synephrine	Sudafed

Diuretics
(used for treatment of edema—swelling of tissues from excess fluids)

Alatone	HydroDIURIL	Regroton
Aldactone	Hydromal	Thalitone
Diuril	Hygroton	Thiuretc
Dyazide	Lasix	
Dyrenium	Midamore	
Esidrix	Oretic	

Muscle relaxants
(used to relieve muscle pain)

Flexeril	Norgesic
Norflex	Paraflex

Stimulants
(used to suppress appetite and in the treatment of certain sleep disorders)

Bimetamphetamine	Dexedrine	Ionamine
Desoxyn	Fastin	

Tranquilizers
(used for control of anxiety and psychotic disorders)

Compazine	Mellaril	Stelazine
Dalmane	Navane	Thorazine
Equanil	Prolixin	Trilafon
Haldol	Serax	Valium
Librium	Sparine	Xanax

HOMEOPATHIC TREATMENT

Dissolve the tablets under your tongue. Do not eat or drink for fifteen minutes prior to or after taking medication. (See Part One, Homeopathy, for additional information.)

Preparation	Directions for Use	Comments
Bryonia 6X	Take 1 tablet 3 times daily.	Indicated for dry mouth and tongue accompanied by cracked lips and excessive thirst.
Natrum muriaticum 30X	Take 1 tablet daily.	Helps improve dry mouth, especially when there are cracks in the corners of the mouth, loss of taste, and dehydration.
X-ray 200X	Take 1 tablet hourly during radiation therapy, then 1 tablet 3 times daily.	Provides relief for dry mouth resulting from radiation therapy.

HERBAL TREATMENT

Herb	Directions for Use	Comments
Aloe vera	Place gel on cotton-tipped swab (see Part Three, Using Herbs, Application Preparation). Apply directly to gums. Do not eat or drink for at least 1 hour after applying the gel.	Soothes dry, inflamed gum tissue.
Eucalyptus oil	Place on a cotton-tipped swab and rub on gums.	Relieves inflamed gums.
Goldenseal	Prepare as a mouthwash (see Part Three, Using Herbs, Mouthwash Preparation). Add 1 teaspoon of baking soda and rinse once a day.	Relieves inflamed gums.

RECOMMENDATIONS

■ Avoid cavity-causing foods—those that contain sugar, those that ferment such as meat and bread, and those that are sticky. Raw vegetables and fruits should be part of your everyday diet. Drink plenty of water and juice to prevent dehydration.

■ Aloe vera gel helps soothe sore gums.

■ *See also* Mouth-Breathing in Part Two.

Dry Socket

Dry socket is the most common complication in wound healing following a tooth extraction. Normally, after a tooth is pulled, a blood clot forms at the base of the socket. If the clot fails to form properly or becomes loose, the exposed tissue and bone can become inflamed and infected. Symptoms of dry socket include radiating, constant pain from the empty tooth socket, swollen gums, fever, and infection. Foul breath, commonly reported as a "bad taste," is another common sign.

CONVENTIONAL TREATMENT

Dry socket heals very slowly because the infection involves the bone. In treating dry socket, the dentist first cleans the area with warm saline and removes any infected bone. A paste made of an antiseptic and analgesic (pain reliever) is placed on a gauze strip, which is then carefully placed in the socket. This dressing is changed daily by the dentist; however, in cases of extreme infection, the dressing may have to be changed two or three times a day. Antibiotics are always prescribed along with pain medication.

NUTRITIONAL SUPPLEMENTS

Supplement	Directions for Use	Comments
Calcium	Take 1500 mg daily.	Important in bone repair.
Garlic	Take 2 capsules of 500 mg each, 3 times daily.	A natural antibiotic and immune system enhancer.
Magnesium	Take 750 mg daily.	Works with calcium to strengthen bone.
Vitamin A + beta-carotene	Take 15,000 IU daily.	Helps heal inflamed tissues and strengthen immune system.
Vitamin C	Take 1500 mg daily.	Promotes healing of infected gums.
Zinc	Take 80 mg daily.	Important in tissue repair.

HOMEOPATHIC TREATMENT

Dissolve the tablets under your tongue. Do not eat or drink for fifteen minutes prior to or after taking medication. (See Part One, Homeopathy, for additional information.)

Preparation	Directions for Use	Comments
Arnica 30X	Take 1 tablet daily.	Helps eliminate bad breath.
Belladonna 6x	Take 1 tablet hourly as needed.	Helps control throbbing pain and fever.
Chamomilla 3X	Take 1 tablet hourly as needed.	Helps control severe pain.
Hepar sulphuris calcareum 6X	Take 1 tablet every 15 minutes as needed.	Helps control bleeding.

HERBAL TREATMENT

Herb	Directions for Use	Comments
Alfalfa	Take 400-mg capsule or tablet form daily.	Helps detoxify the blood.

Echinacea	Take 450-mg capsule or tablet every 2 hours. Decrease as needed.	Has antibiotic and anti-inflammatory properties.
Goldenseal	Take 400-mg capsule or tablet daily.	Strengthens immune system; has antibiotic and anti-inflammatory properties.
Horsetail	Take 400-mg capsule or tablet daily.	Accelerates healing of wounds.

RECOMMENDATIONS

■   For the initial forty-five to sixty minutes following the removal of a tooth, it is critical to keep the area clean to promote clot formation. The best way to do this is by biting on a clean piece of gauze for at least forty-five minutes following the extraction. (The gauze is usually placed in the area by the dentist before you leave the office.)

■   Do not suck on a straw, spit, smoke, touch the area with a tongue or finger, or eat for at least three hours following a tooth extraction. These actions may cause delayed clotting or contamination of the area, which may result in dry socket.

SOURCES OF HELP

There are groups to which those suffering from anorexia or bulimia can turn for help:

American Anorexia/Bulimia Association (AABA)
293 Central Park West
Suite 1R
New York, NY 10024
212–501–8351

Anorexia Nervosa and Related Eating Disorders (ANRED)
P.O. Box 5102
Eugene, OR 97405
503–344–1144

Institute for the Study of Anorexia and Bulimia
1 West 91 Street
New York, NY 10024
212–595–3449

National Association of Anorexia Nervosa and Associated Disorders
P.O. Box 7
Highland Park, IL 60035
708–831–3438

National Eating Disorders Organization (NEDO)
445 East Granville Road
Worthington, OH 43085–3195
614–436–1112

Eating Disorders and Tooth Problems

Anorexia nervosa and bulimia are two serious eating disorders that, among other conditions, can result in tooth problems. Adolescent and twenty- to thirty-year-old females are particularly at risk of developing an eating disorder, though males can be affected as well.

Anorexia nervosa is characterized by an inordinate fear of gaining weight. Starvation, use of laxatives, and self-induced vomiting lead to weight loss and, eventually, malnutrition. Bulimia is characterized by an unsatisfied yearning for food. A bulimic person engages in a secret cycle of eating binges that are followed by self-induced vomiting to rid the body of the consumed calories.

Because the stomach acid from frequent vomiting leads to severe erosion of tooth enamel, a dentist may be the first to notice the signs of such eating disorders. Teeth will appear worn and yellow. Other symptoms may include irritation of the throat and esophagus, chest pain, and salivary gland swelling.

CONVENTIONAL TREATMENT

A dentist can diagnose the condition and correct the deteriorated tooth enamel with cosmetic dentistry, but he or she cannot treat the actual eating disorder. Anorexia and bulimia are potentially life-threatening conditions that revolve around issues of self-image and self-control. Treatment requires addressing of the psychological issues while restoring and maintaining nutritional needs.

RECOMMENDATIONS

- Get help by contacting one of the organizations listed in the margin.
- *See also* Cosmetic Dentistry in Part Three.

Emergencies, Dental

See First Aid in Part Three for specific information on dealing with such common dental emergencies as severe toothaches; breaking of a crown, bridge, or tooth; loss of a filling; and mouth pain from erupting teeth, surgery, or orthodontia.

See also Braces-Related Problems; Bridge-Related Problems; Wisdom-Teeth-Related Problems in Part Two.

Endodontic Problems

The term "endodontic problems" refers to those conditions associated with the tooth root, dental pulp, and surrounding tissue. There are numerous causes of these problems. Bacteria present in deep cavities or gum disease may infect or kill the pulp tissue. This is usually the result of failure to have routine dental checkups or of poor oral hygiene. Sometimes, ill-fitting crowns and fillings may be responsible for bacteria reaching the pulp tissue. Also, certain chemicals found in some filling materials and cements may be toxic to pulp tissue. In other instances injury and trauma caused by tooth fracture may damage or kill pulp tissue. If a cavity is deep enough to affect the area containing the nerve and blood supply, or if a gum abscess affects the area, root canal therapy is called for. In both situations, pain is experienced when heat, cold, or pressure is applied to the affected tooth. Other symptoms of endodontic problems include gum swelling around the root of a tooth, and tenderness and/or swelling in glands under the jaw.

CONVENTIONAL TREATMENT

Root canal therapy (see Endodontic Techniques in Part Three) is performed to treat diseased or damaged tooth pulp. When the therapy is performed properly, the success rate is very high, and the tooth is saved, preventing extraction. Contrary to the fears of most individuals, root canal treatment is not a painful procedure. Once a local anesthetic is given, the patient feels no pain during the procedure. Sometimes, if the infection is severe, the anesthetic may not allow the tooth to become adequately anesthetized. In this case, antibiotic and pain medication is given, and the person returns for the root canal therapy when the infection has subsided.

89

A number of dentists perform root canal treatments if they feel there is even a chance that such treatment is required. Other dentists first try treating the tooth with a material containing a mixture of clove oil and zinc oxide and wait for the tooth's response. Sometimes, the tooth heals after this material is placed in a tooth, and root canal therapy may not be required. If the nerve is not damaged too severely, any pain will decrease within three days. The paste is usually left in the tooth for six weeks, and then a permanent filling or crown is placed on the tooth. During the six weeks, the dentin is able to regenerate secondary dentin over the deep areas where the cavity had been. If an x-ray reveals an infection, then root canal therapy or extraction of the tooth is the only option. A decision has to be made quickly as to the treatment of choice. If gum disease in the form of bone loss is present, or if the infection is extensive and has caused bone loss, tooth extraction may be the best option.

NUTRITIONAL SUPPLEMENTS

Supplement	Directions for Use	Comments
Garlic	Take two 250-mg tablets 3 times daily.	A natural antibiotic; protects against infection.
Kelp	Take 500 mg daily.	An important source of trace minerals; helps maintain healthy bones and gums.
Vitamin A	Take 20,000 IU daily.	Enhances tissue healing.
Vitamin B complex	Take 100 mg daily.	Important in stress management.
Vitamin C	Take 2000 mg daily.	Helps promote healing.

HOMEOPATHIC TREATMENT

Dissolve the tablets under your tongue. Do not eat or drink for fifteen minutes prior to or after taking medication. (See Part One, Homeopathy, for additional information.)

Preparation	Directions for Use	Comments
Belladonna 30X	Take 1 tablet hourly.	For relief of toothache and pain associated with abscess.
Chamomilla 30X	Take 1 tablet hourly.	For relief of severe tooth pain in response to heat.
Hypericum 30X	Take 1 tablet 3 times daily.	Helps repair nerve tissue.

HERBAL TREATMENT

Herb	Directions for Use	Comments
Peppermint oil	Place on a cotton-tipped swab and apply to the aching tooth.	Helps relieve tooth pain.

| Alfalfa | Prepare as a tea (see Part Three, Using Herbs, Tea Preparation) and drink 2–3 cups daily, or take capsules or tablets as directed on package. | An excellent blood purifier, supplies vital trace minerals. |
| Red clover | Prepare as a tea (see Part Three, Using Herbs, Tea Preparation) and drink 2–3 cups daily, or take capsules or tablets as directed on package. | An excellent blood purifier. |

RECOMMENDATIONS

■ It may be advantageous to seek treatment from a specialist rather than a general dentist, in case complications occur. An endodontist is trained to perform root canal therapy.

■ If there is any question regarding the need for root canal therapy, the dentist should attempt to treat the tooth first with a mixture of clove oil and zinc oxide (see Conventional Treatment, above).

■ Do not eat hot or cold foods right after root canal treatment, and do not chew hard foods with the affected tooth.

Extraction, Tooth.

See Tooth Extraction in Part Three.

Facial Pain

See TMJ.

Facial Paralysis

The face may become paralyzed due to strokes, tumors, viruses, or severe trauma to the head area that severs certain facial nerves. Usually, half of the face is affected, with the eye having a tendency to roll upward, as seen in Bell's palsy. The person will be unable to open the eyelid on the paralyzed side, the lip will sag, and he or she will be unable to smile or wrinkle the forehead. Taste and hearing may also be altered.

Exposure to draft, upper respiratory infections, or administration of routine dental anesthetic can sometimes cause Bell's palsy, paralysis of any or all branches of the facial nerve that controls the muscles of the face. Bell's palsy may occur suddenly; some patients have reported discovering the paralysis upon waking. Others have reported pain around the ear and face for a few days prior to the onset of paralysis. The paralysis may be incomplete and temporary, with recovery occurring in three to six weeks. If there is partial nerve damage, improvement is noted no later than twelve weeks after the initial symptoms. Eighty to eighty-five percent of patients with Bell's palsy recover fully or almost so. In a smaller percentage of people, persistent facial weakness, uncontrollable eye winking, or excessive tearing continues.

Sometimes, paralysis occurs after an anesthetic is accidentally injected into the parotid gland. The paralysis usually wears off a few hours after the injection is administered. In some cases, the paralysis causes a permanent disability, and there is no improvement even after three or more months.

Trigeminal neuralgia or tic douloureux is a disorder of unknown cause that affects one or both of the trigeminal nerves, the largest pair of nerves in the skull, serving most of the face including the jaws. Symptoms include severe, stabbing pain that may last seconds to minutes. Often, the pain occurs on one side of the face and is usually accompanied by muscle spasms.

CONVENTIONAL TREATMENT

If paralysis is complete from the beginning, the patient is observed carefully. Approximately one week after the onset of the paralysis, electrodiagnostic tests are performed to determine the extent of damage to the nerves. Prednisone (a steroid used to treat inflammation and prevent allergic reaction) is usually recommended as soon as possible to decrease the effects of the paralysis. Severe paralysis has distressing cosmetic effects. Surgery to connect and activate some of the nerves may be helpful. Pain medications may also be prescribed. For trigeminal neuralgia, Tegretol, an anticonvulsant used mostly for epilepsy, is prescribed.

NUTRITIONAL SUPPLEMENTS

Supplement	Directions for Use	Comments
Calcium	Take 1500 mg daily.	Important for proper nerve transmission and muscle function.
Coenzyme Q-10	Take 60 mg daily.	Improves circulation and transport of oxygen.
Magnesium	Take 750 mg daily.	Works in conjunction with calcium in nerve and muscle function.
Vitamin B_1	Take 100 mg daily.	Involved in release of energy in muscles and nerves.
Vitamin E	Take 400 IU daily.	As an antioxidant, may be important to the healing process.

HOMEOPATHIC TREATMENT

Dissolve the tablets under your tongue. Do not eat or drink for fifteen minutes prior to or after taking medication. (See Part One, Homeopathy, for additional information.)

Preparation	Directions for Use	Comments
Aconite 6X	Take 1 tablet hourly.	Indicated for relief from numbness and anxiety.
Ammonium phosphoricum 3X	Take 1 tablet daily.	Helps relieve symptoms of facial paralysis.
Causticum 30X	Take 1 tablet hourly or daily as needed.	Recommended to help relieve pain associated with facial paralysis.
Dulcamara 30X	Take 1 tablet 3 times daily.	Indicated when draft causes the paralysis to become worse.

HERBAL TREATMENT

Herb	Directions for Use	Comments
Black cohosh, catnip, red clover, and yellow dock	Prepare together as tea (see Part Three, Using Herbs, Tea Preparation). Drink as needed for relaxation.	Catnip has a sedative effect; black cohosh is an antispasmodic; clover and yellow dock are tonics.
Goldenseal	Take 400-mg tablets 3 times daily.	For relief of pain of facial paralysis.
Skullcap	Take 400-mg tablets 3 times daily.	For relief of pain of facial paralysis.

RECOMMENDATONS

■ During paralysis, control of the facial muscles is lost, and the delicate cornea may be accidentally damaged. Wearing an eyepad may help protect the cornea.

■ Massaging the affected muscles to promote circulation may help the healing process.

■ A splint made by the dentist may help with droopy facial muscles.

Fillings, Loss of

See First Aid in Part Three.

Finger-Biting-Related Dental Problems

A common habit among both children and adults, nail- and/or finger-biting damages the nails and can also damage the teeth and jaw joint. Any habit that involves holding the tooth in an abnormal position for prolonged periods of time can eventually cause problems in the jaw joint (*see* TMJ in Part Two). If nail- and/or finger-biting is a long-term habit, it will stretch the muscles in the jaw, causing pain and an imbalance in the joints. If the habit begins when a child is very young, it can cause a gap between the front teeth. People who bite their fingers and nails may also pick at their gums, causing damage to that tissue.

CONVENTIONAL TREATMENT

Each dentist or physician has a favorite treatment to stop nail- and finger-biting. Some recommend putting bitter-tasting substances such as pepper or nontoxic lotions on the fingers. Others tie a bow around or put a bandage on the finger to serve as a reminder.

Orthodontic treatment will be required to close any gap between teeth caused by nail- or finger-biting. Jaw joint problems may have to be addressed (see TMJ in Part Two).

NUTRITIONAL SUPPLEMENTS

Supplement	Directions for Use	Comments
Calcium	Take 1500 mg daily.	Due to its relationship to the nervous system and the muscles, it has a calming effect.
Magnesium	Take 750 mg daily.	Works in conjunction with calcium in nerve function.
Vitamin B complex	Take 50 mg daily.	Important for function of nervous system; considered an "anti-stress" vitamin.

HOMEOPATHIC TREATMENT

Dissolve the tablets under your tongue. Do not eat or drink for fifteen minutes prior to or after taking medication. (See Part One, Homeopathy, for additional information.)

Preparation	Directions for Use	Comments
Aconite 30X	Take 1 tablet 3 times a day.	Helps allay anxiety, fear, and physical and mental restlessness.
Ambra grisia 3X	Take 1 tablet daily.	Indicated for children with extreme nervousness.

HERBAL TREATMENT

Herb	Directions for Use	Comments
Chamomile	Prepare as tea (see Part Three, Using Herbs, Tea Preparation). Drink 2–3 cups daily.	Promotes relaxation.
Lobelia	Prepare as tea (see Part Three, Using Herbs, Tea Preparation). Drink 2–3 cups daily.	A powerful relaxant.

RECOMMENDATIONS

■ A positive way of breaking the nail- or finger-biting habit in children is to do the following: Keep a record of days that your child has not bitten his or her nails or fingers by marking the days with stars on a calendar. At the end of a certain number of days in a row without nail- or finger-biting (number of days to be determined by you), the child should get a reward. If the fingers or nails are bitten, the stars must be started again from day one.

■ During the day, place a bandage on the finger as a reminder not to bite it.

■ Among adults, regular professional manicures have been reported to be a safe way to break the habit. The desire to bite fingers or nails is diminished when the nails are kept clean and trimmed by a manicurist.

■ *See also* TMJ in Part Two; and Orthodontic Techniques in Part Three.

Fluoride-Related Tooth Problems

Researchers in the 1930s found that people who grew up drinking naturally fluoridated water had up to two-thirds less cavities than people living in areas without fluoridated water. In 1945, researchers added fluoride to the drinking water in Newburgh, New York and Grand Rapids, Michigan, and soon discovered that tooth decay decreased in these cities. By the 1950s, public health officials were recommending fluoridation of water in all communities.

The World Health Organization, the American Dental Association, and the American Medical Association have endorsed the use of fluoride in water supplies because of its effect on dental caries. The main component of tooth enamel is hydroxyapatite, a very porous crystalline structure. Fluoride fills in the holes in the structure, making the enamel more resistant to acid and, therefore, to cavities. It has also been suggested that fluoride may decrease the pH of plaque, making it less able to cause gum damage and cavities. Health organizations believe this benefit involves little or no risk and argue that fluoridation is more cost-effective than the high cost of dental treatment for decayed teeth. Nevertheless, many people feel health matters are a personal choice and they should not be forced to drink fluoridated water.

DID YOU KNOW . . .

Fluorine (F) is a poisonous and highly corrosive gas. It belongs to the halogen group of chemicals, which includes chlorine, bromine, iodine, and astatine. Fluorine is important largely because of its compounds, which include fluoride and fluorocarbons. The latter are used extensively in lubricants and bearings because of their low friction. The best known of the fluorocarbons is probably Teflon.

When deciding whether water should be fluoridated, people must consider the benefits and risks. In most countries other than the United States, fluoridation is not used. Fluoride, a compound of fluorine, is a common element in the Earth's crust, and is widely distributed in nature. Almost all foods and water supplies contain some fluoride; there are 1.8466 billion tons of sodium fluoride in the oceans, and marine life is exposed to 1.3 parts fluoride per million parts of water. Fluoride is also found in vegetables, depending on the amount found in the water used to irrigate the soil.

The safe level of fluoridated water is 1 ppm (part per million). As the levels of fluoride increase to 2 or 3 ppm and above, damage to bone and the teeth is seen. The teeth may appear discolored and somewhat chalky looking (mottled) with higher levels of fluoridation. Mottling may sometimes be observed even with accepted levels of fluoride in water. And fluoride uptake by the kidneys may present a risk for individuals with kidney disease.

Once absorbed, fluoride concentrates in bones and teeth. What is not absorbed is excreted in urine and sweat, and in the milk of nursing mothers. The heaviest fluoride deposits occur in the growing bones and developing teeth of children under the age of nine. Fluoride concentration in enamel increases until a person is thirty to forty years of age, and then levels off. Pediatricians and pediatric dentists recommend fluoride drops for infants age six months and older when the water supply does not have fluoride. They also recommend fluoride supplements for children who get many cavities or who have medical conditions that make proper hygiene impossible. In such cases, fluoride may also be applied in the dentist's office. (See Fluoride Treatment in Part Three.)

Many mouthwashes and toothpastes contain fluoride. Those containing stannous fluoride have a bitter taste and tend to stain the teeth temporarily. Sodium monofluorophosphate is commonly used in toothpastes because it is stable at a variety of pH levels and is well absorbed by the body. Calcium fluoride is not very soluble and, therefore, may actually cause calcium ions to form around the teeth, leading to tartar build-up. Most studies have shown that using toothpaste that contains fluoride is not effective in decay prevention. Rather, proper oral hygiene and diet are the most reliable means of preventing tooth decay.

CONVENTIONAL TREATMENT

Mottling is the only dental problem related to fluoride use. Treatment may include covering the teeth with cosmetic porcelain veneers, bleaching the teeth, or gently abrading the outer layer of enamel that shows the mottling. (See Cosmetic Dentistry in Part Three.)

RECOMMENDATIONS

■ Generally speaking, bottled water—with or without fluoride—may be safer to drink than the water in many communities. The mineral content and contamination of many public water supplies may vary from day to day.

■ You can remove fluoride and toxins from your water supply with a reverse osmosis and/or distillation systems.

■ *See also* Fluoride Treatment in Part Three.

Fracture, Jaw

See Jaw Fracture.

Fracture, Tooth

See Broken, Cracked, or Chipped Teeth.

Gingivitis

See Gum Disease.

Glossitis

See Tongue-Related Problems.

Grinding, Tooth

See Bruxism.

Gum Disease

The gum tissue that surrounds the teeth is called gingiva. The gingiva, the bones forming the tooth socket, and the supporting ligaments are referred to collectively as periodontium. Gum or periodontal disease refers to a variety of problems affecting the gums and bone that hold the teeth in place. These problems include bleeding, swelling, receding gums, and loose teeth. Nearly 85 percent of the

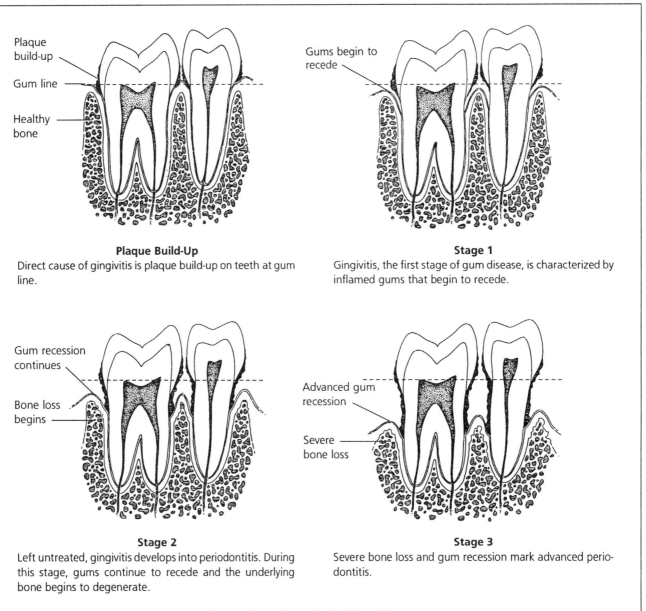

Plaque Build-Up
Direct cause of gingivitis is plaque build-up on teeth at gum line.

Stage 1
Gingivitis, the first stage of gum disease, is characterized by inflamed gums that begin to recede.

Stage 2
Left untreated, gingivitis develops into periodontitis. During this stage, gums continue to recede and the underlying bone begins to degenerate.

Stage 3
Severe bone loss and gum recession mark advanced periodontitis.

Progression of Periodontal (Gum) Disease

population has some form of this disease. Since there is no pain or discomfort present during the initial stages, people often ignore the signs and symptoms, believing them to be normal occurrences. For example, some bleeding during brushing and flossing, or loosening of teeth as one gets older is taken for granted. Knowledge about gum disease is, therefore, imperative to dental health.

Healthy gums are firm and springy, and vary in color depending on the thickness of the outer layer. A change in normal color is one of the first signs of gum disease, which has three stages: gingivitis, periodontitis, and advanced periodontitis (pyorrhea). This progression is illustrated by the figures above.

Gingivitis—an inflammation of the gums—is the initial stage of gum disease and the easiest to treat. The direct cause of gingivitis is plaque—the soft, sticky, almost colorless film that forms continuously on the teeth and gums. Plaque is not harmful

8 Ways to Stop Bleeding Gums

Bleeding gums are often a sign of gum disease. It is important to do something immediately to remedy the situation. The following are eight effective ways to treat bleeding gums.

1. Floss daily. Plaque build-up is a major cause of gum disease. Flossing not only keeps plaque from building on teeth, it also prevents it from building on gums. (For more information on proper flossing techniques, see Oral Hygiene, Flossing, in Part Three.)

2. Brush properly after every meal to remove food particles. (For more information on proper brushing techniques, see Oral Hygiene, Brushing, in Part Three.)

3. Consider using an electric toothbrush, which is effective in stimulating and cleaning gums.

4. Have your teeth cleaned and checked regularly by a dental hygienist, dentist, or periodontist.

5. To soothe and heal inflamed, bleeding gums, rinse your mouth with a solution of warm water mixed with a tablespoon of aloe vera gel, or apply aloe vera gel directly to the affected area. (See Using Herbs, Application Preparation, in Part Three.)

6. Use goldenseal in a toothpaste preparation to help heal inflamed, diseased gums. (See Using Herbs, Application Preparation, in Part Three.)

7. Vitamin C is important for healthy gums. Take the recommended adult requirement of 500 milligrams daily.

8. For gums that have receded, use balsa-wood wedge toothpicks to clean between the gums and teeth. (For further information on these special toothpicks, see Oral Hygiene in Part Three.) Do not use regular toothpicks, which may damage delicate gum tissue and wear down the sides of the teeth causing "toothpick abrasion."

if it is removed before it begins to accumulate. However, if teeth and gums are not cleaned thoroughly every twenty-four to thirty-six hours, the bacteria in plaque produce toxins and enzymes that inflame the gums. Due to this inflammation, the gums become slightly red and puffy and may bleed during brushing or flossing; the gums may also begin to recede (pull away) slightly from the tooth or teeth. During this early stage of gum disease, called gingivitis, damage can be reversed since the bone and connective tissue that hold the teeth in place are not yet affected.

Other factors that may contribute to gingivitis include habitual clenching and grinding of the teeth (see Bruxism in Part Two) and mouth-breathing (see Dry Mouth; Mouth-Breathing-Related Problems in Part Two). A diet that is high in simple carbohydrates and sugar and deficient in vitamins also contributes to gingivitis, as well as the use of tobacco, drugs, and alcohol. Heredity, hormonal imbalances (during pregnancy and puberty), oral contraceptives, and stress are other possible contributors.

If gingivitis is left untreated, the inflammation can spread to the roots of the teeth developing into periodontitis. During this second stage of gum disease, the plaque penetrates deeper into the gum tissues and eventually begins to affect the under-lying bone. As the disease continues to advance, the gums further recede from the teeth giving them an elongated appearance. Gum pockets form, in which more

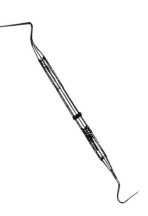

Periodontal Probe
Used to measure depth of
gum pocket.

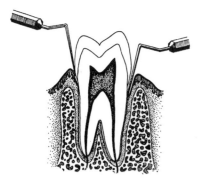

**Measuring Depth
of Gum Pocket**
At left, periodontal probe
measures depth of healthy
gum. At right, probe measures
deep pocket in unhealthy gum.

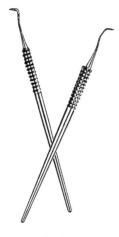

Scalers
Used to scrape plaque and
tartar off tooth surfaces.

plaque and food debris collects. These pockets prevent easy cleaning and elimination of plaque under the gums, causing halitosis (see Bad Breath in Part Two) and pain. Accumulation of bacteria causes infections that begin to destroy the bone. Abscesses (see Abscesses in Part Two) may form, the teeth may shift or become loose, and the bite may change. Tartar or mineralized plaque deposits further irritate the gums. Any pressure on the gums during this stage may cause heavy bleeding or the discharge of pus.

The third stage of gum disease, advanced periodontitis or pyorrhea, is marked by major gum recession and severe bone loss. At this point, the teeth are often too loose to be saved and frequently have to be pulled.

Acute necrotizing ulcerative gingivitis (ANUG), also called Vincent's disease or trench mouth, is another type of gum disease. Symptoms of ANUG include ulcers along the gum line and between the teeth. It is often accompanied by fever, swollen glands, nausea, headaches, and general weakness. Although ANUG appears suddenly, its causative factors—poor oral hygiene, physical and mental stress, weakened immune system due to illness—usually have been present for some time.

CONVENTIONAL TREATMENT

The only effective long-term treatment of gum disease is to deal with its underlying causes and to keep the teeth and gums clean. Good oral hygiene includes regular professional cleanings. Such cleanings are extremely important at the first sign of gingivitis.

Be aware that each stage of gum disease requires a different type of cleaning. For early-stage gingivitis, a one-time professional cleaning is usually sufficient. During this visit (as well as visits for more advanced gum disease), a periodontal probe (see margin figure) will be used to determine the degree of gum damage. One end of the probe has bands that indicate millimeters. This end is gently placed between the tooth and gum to measure gum pocket depth (see margin figure). For healthy gums, pocket depth is from 2 and 3 millimeters. As mild to moderate pain may be felt during the cleaning, your dentist may first numb the area with a topical anesthetic. After the cleaning, you will probably be asked to return in three months for a check-up and another routine cleaning. If the gums appear healthy at that point, you will likely be asked to either continue the three-month recalls or return in four to six months.

Periodontitis and advanced periodontitis require more than a routine cleaning. Bacteria has caused a build-up of plaque and tartar deep into the gum tissue and on the tooth root. Scalers (see margin figure) are used to scrape plaque and tartar off the surface of the teeth (scaling), including the roots (root planing). Plaque and infected tissue are removed from the walls of the gum pockets (curettage). Depending on the extent of the infection, the amount of plaque and tartar, and the depth of the pockets, the procedure may require one or more visits. Local anesthetic may be used during this procedure if the pain is severe. Antibiotics may be prescribed if abscesses are present.

Your dentist may refer you to a periodontist for deep-cleanings or for surgery to remove diseased gum tissue and to reshape the bone. However, surgery will not bring about a permanent cure unless the cause of the disease is determined and eliminated. In the case of advanced periodontitis, splinting the teeth (holding several teeth in place by means of a wire, plastic, or resin material) and bone and gum grafting may be considered instead of tooth extraction.

NUTRITIONAL SUPPLEMENTS

Supplement	Directions for Use	Comments
Calcium	Take 1500 mg daily.	Important component of strong, healthy bones.
Coenzyme Q-10	Take 60 mg daily.	Helps improve gum disease by increasing circulation of oxygen to cells.
Garlic	Take 250 mg daily.	Nature's antibiotic. Also helps strengthen the immune system.
Magnesium	Take 750 mg daily.	Works with calcium in maintaining healthy bones.
Vitamin A	Take 10,000 IU daily.	Helps fight infection.
Vitamin B complex	Take 100 mg daily.	Involved in the production of energy through the conversion of food. Beneficial effect on stress.
Vitamin C	Take 1500 mg daily.	An important component of connective tissue; promotes healing of bleeding, unhealthy gums.
Zinc	Take 60 mg daily.	Promotes healing.

HOMEOPATHIC TREATMENT

Dissolve the tablets under your tongue. Do not eat or drink for fifteen minutes prior to or after taking medication. (See Part One, Homeopathy, for additional information.)

Preparation	Directions for Use	Comments
Kali phosphoricum 6X	Take 1 tablet 3 times daily or every 2 hours, depending on the severity of the problem.	Helpful for gums that bleed easily and for spongy, receding gums.
Mercurius corrrosivus 6X	Take 1 tablet 3 times daily.	Indicated for loose teeth and swollen gums.
Mercurius hydrargyrum 30X	Take 1 tablet 3 times daily.	Helps stop bleeding; heals receding, tender gums; and alleviates bad breath.

HERBAL TREATMENT

Herb	Directions for Use	Comments
Aloe vera	Place gel on a cotton-tipped swab (see Part Three, Using Herbs, Application Preparation). Apply to gums at bedtime.	Helps soothe and heal sore, inflamed gums.
Goldenseal	Prepare as toothpaste (see Part Three, Using Herbs, Application Preparation). Brush 3 times a day.	Helps heal gum disease.

✍ TAKE NOTE . . .

Electric toothbrushes are designed so that the bristles move within the head of the brush, while the head and handle remain stationary. This produces quick, short vibrating strokes that do a superior job in cleaning teeth and stimulating gums.

There are many electric toothbrush systems on the market. However, they are not all the same. The Interplak system has stiff bristles that vibrate rapidly. Oral B and Braun system toothbrushes have round heads and soft bristles. Some systems brush the tongue side and the cheek side of the teeth at the same time.

The Rododent system, which is not available in stores, is a superior electric toothbrush. The head is small and round, and shaped like the polishing tool the dentist or hygienist uses after scaling the teeth. The bristles are soft, causing minimal abrasion. The Rododent system also comes with a pointed brush to clean between teeth, bridges, braces, and other hard-to-reach areas. The instructions recommend that you brush each tooth for just one second with this system.

In general, choose an electric toothbrush that has a full tuft of soft bristles that rotates gently. It's also important to choose a brush with a small head that cleans one tooth surface at a time.

For information on water irrigating devices, see Oral Hygiene in Part Three.

RECOMMENDATIONS

■ Avoid mouthwashes that contain alcohol; they may irritate and dry gum tissues.

■ If a gum infection exists, use a 3 percent hydrogen peroxide solution (available at any pharmacy) as a rinse; it will help destroy bacteria and clean the gum tissues. However, long-term use of hydrogen peroxide is not recommended as it may eventually destroy delicate gum tissue, leaving a whitish patch behind.

■ Toothpaste with aloe vera and baking soda (Grace, for example) is more soothing to the gum tissues than pastes with harsh chemicals.

■ Consider using an electric toothbrush system (see margin note), which many dentists feel is very effective in cleaning teeth and stimulating gums.

■ Avoid spicy foods, foods that are high in sugar, and meats. Because healing is promoted by proper nutrition, eat a balanced diet that includes raw and steamed vegetables and fruits. Drink adequate amounts of water—at least eight 8-ounce glasses each day—because bacteria tend to thrive in a dry environment. Because of their high sugar content, avoid soft drinks and sodas.

■ Medications such as Dilantin, which is used for control of epilepsy, and Inderol, used for hypertension and heart disease, may cause inflammation and swelling of the gums. If proper hygiene does not control the swelling, your physician may need to reduce the dosage or prescribe a substitute.

■ *See also* Gum Surgery in Part Three.

Gums, Bleeding

See Gum Disease.

Gums, Receding

Receding gums exist when the gums and the bone have moved away from the tooth. This may be caused by gum disease (see Gum Disease in Part Two), imbalanced occlusion, or trauma. Accumulation of plaque at the gum line and poor oral hygiene also lead to receding gums. Bacteria in the plaque release toxic fluids that cause destruction of gum tissue.

When occlusion (the way the teeth come together) is imbalanced, excessive forces placed on the teeth cause trauma to the bone and gums. The result is resorption of bone and recession of the gums. Gum recession exposes the roots, causing the teeth to become sensitive to hot, cold, sweet, and salty substances.

Excessive pressure resulting from grinding or clenching teeth may cause the gums to recede. Receding gums are also in evidence when teeth are crooked, or fillings and crowns are placed without properly balancing the bite. In both of these cases, the teeth do not come together properly, and increased forces placed on certain parts of the teeth cause delicate fibers around the gums to become crushed and torn. Some people falsely think that brushing the teeth too vigorously causes receding gums. Brushing vigorously increases sensitivity in the area as exposed root surfaces become abraded; however, it does not cause receding gums.

Initially, the gums and bone adjust to excessive forces; however, if the forces continue, resorption of bone results. Because the teeth and the supporting structures have the ability to adapt, you may not realize gum recession is occurring until you notice sensitivity or see the changes around the teeth.

CONVENTIONAL TREATMENT

Receded gums are initially reversible; however, over the long term, they will not return to normal. Correcting the cause of the recession will prevent further damage. Fillings and crowns that do not meet properly should be corrected, and grinding and clenching the teeth should be stopped.

Once the gums have receded, the teeth may become sensitive. Your dentist may prescribe fluoride to be applied to the sensitive areas or to be used as a rinse. It is not clear why the fluoride is effective, but a paste consisting of equal parts of sodium fluoride, kaolin, and glycerin; a solution of 2 percent sodium silicofluoride; and a 1-percent solution of sodium fluoride have all been used successfully on sensitive areas of teeth where the gums have receded. Other agents used for desensitizing teeth are parachlorophenol, metacresyl acetate (Cresatin), gum camphor, and prednisone. Most of these agents are in solution form and are applied to the sensitive area with a cotton swab. Special toothpastes such as Sensodyne, Denquile, and Grace are also helpful. If the teeth continue to be sensitive, composite resins or other types of fillings, such as amalgam or gold, may be placed in the tooth.

NUTRITIONAL SUPPLEMENTS

Supplement	Directions for Use	Comments
Calcium	Take 1200 mg daily.	Helps maintain healthy bones and teeth.
Magnesium	Take 600 mg daily.	Works with calcium as an important part of healthy bones and teeth. Helps prevent bone loss.
Phosphorus	Take 1200 mg daily.	Helps prevent decay on exposed dentin.
Vitamin B complex	Take 100 mg daily.	Helps manage stress.
Vitamin C	Take 1500 mg daily.	Important for repair of gum tissue.

HOMEOPATHIC TREATMENT

Dissolve the tablets under your tongue. Do not eat or drink for fifteen minutes prior to or after taking medication. (See Part One, Homeopathy, for additional information.)

Preparation	Directions for Use	Comments
Plantago major 6X	Take 1 tablet 3 times daily.	Relieves sensitivity of teeth to cold and pressure.
Silicea 6X	Take 1 tablet daily.	Relieves sensitivity of teeth to cold.

HERBAL TREATMENT

Preparation	Directions for Use	Comments
Myrrh	Prepare as a mouthwash (see Part Three, Using Herbs, Mouthwash Preparation). Use as needed.	Gives instant, temporary relief to toothache.
Peppermint, clove oil	Prepare the herbs together or separately as a mouthwash (see Part Three, Using Herbs, Mouthwash Preparation). Use as needed.	Relieves toothache pain.

RECOMMENDATIONS

■ Determining and treating the cause of gum recession will prevent it from getting worse.

■ *See also* Gum Disease in Part Two; and Oral Hygiene in Part Three.

Halitosis

See Bad Breath.

Headaches, Dental-Related

See Migraine Headache; TMJ.

Herpes Simplex

See Oral Herpes Infection.

Herpetic Stomatitis

See Oral Herpes Infection.

Impacted Teeth

Sometimes, teeth do not erupt. They may be impacted for a variety of reasons such as crowding, cysts, or other unknown causes. Wisdom teeth, the third molars and the last teeth to erupt, may not develop at all or may be impacted within the jawbone. In this case, they cannot erupt properly and may have to be surgically removed. Sometimes, teeth other than the third molars become impacted. When possible, these teeth are not removed, but are helped to erupt normally. See figure below for illustration of impacted teeth.

CONVENTIONAL TREATMENT

If possible, an oral surgeon exposes an impacted primary or secondary tooth. The orthodontist then brings the tooth to its proper position with braces. If a person's jaw is too small to allow the tooth to grow properly, the impacted tooth is surgically removed. Approximately 25 percent of the people who have impacted teeth extracted develop dry socket (see Dry Socket in Part Two).

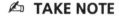 **TAKE NOTE**

Impacted teeth can cause inflammation of surrounding tissue, which may lead to infection. Be sure to see your dentist if the gum tissues become red, inflamed, and painful.

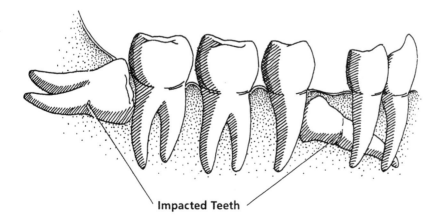

Impacted Teeth

NUTRITIONAL SUPPLEMENTS

Supplement	Directions for Use	Comments
Calcium	Take 800 mg daily.	Important for development of healthy bone.
Magnesium	Take 400 mg daily.	Aids calcium assimilation.
Vitamin C	Take 200 mg daily.	For relief of sore gums surrounding impacted teeth.

HOMEOPATHIC TREATMENT

Dissolve the tablets under your tongue. Do not eat or drink for fifteen minutes prior to or after taking medication. (See Part One, Homeopathy, for additional information.)

Preparation	Directions for Use	Comments
Belladonna 30X	Take 1 tablet 3 times a day.	Indicated for fever and pain associated with erupting teeth.
Chamomilla 30X	Take 1 tablet hourly.	Helps heal irritated gums surrounding impacted or erupting teeth.

HERBAL TREATMENT

Herb	Directions for Use	Comments
Aloe vera	Prepare as a mouthwash (see Part Three, Using Herbs, Mouthwash Preparation) and rinse at bedtime. Or place gel on a cotton-tipped swab (see Part Three, Using Herbs, Application Preparation) and rub on gums.	Relieves inflamed gums.
Eucalyptus oil	Place on a cotton-tipped swab and rub on gums.	Helps heal irritated gums surrounding impacted or erupting teeth.

RECOMMENDATIONS

■ Whenever possible, impacted teeth should be exposed and brought into proper position as soon as possible.

■ Warm salt-water rinses are helpful when the area surrounding an impacted tooth becomes sore and infected.

■ *See also* Wisdom-Teeth-Related Problems in Part Two; and Tooth Extraction in Part Three.

Infection

As with any part of the body, if the mouth is invaded by a particular type of bacteria, virus, or fungus, the toxins generated by the microorganism may cause an infection. The mouth is inhabited by many microorganisms. However, if an environment is produced in which a certain type of microorganism will overwhelmingly grow and multiply, then an infection may result.

With proper hygiene and a healthy immune system, the microorganisms present in the mouth will be harmless. If the immune system is not healthy, the ability to resist illness is compromised. Sometimes, drugs and disease reduce a person's immunity, and sometimes the microorganism itself may be particularly virulent or toxic.

Infection related to the gums, the teeth, or any other part of the mouth is accompanied by redness, swelling, and pain. When an abscess is present, there is a localized collection of pus. (See Abscess in Part Two.) If the infection spreads to surrounding tissues, it is called cellulitis. Bacteria can sometimes be found in normally sterile blood (bacteremia), or the infection can become systemic, disseminating organisms throughout the blood stream (septicemia).

CONVENTIONAL TREATMENT

A dentist first determines the cause of the infection and then administers appropriate treatment, which may involve pulling an infected tooth, draining a gum abscess and cleaning the gums thoroughly, or performing root canal treatment. Antibiotics are given for bacterial infection, and drugs are prescribed for pain. Hospitalization may be required for severe infections that have spread.

NUTRITIONAL SUPPLEMENTS

Supplement	Directions for Use	Comments
Coenzyme Q-10	Take 60 mg daily.	By improving circulation, it improves transport of oxygen to gum tissues, which is important in the healing process.
Garlic	Take two 250-mg tablets 3 times a day.	Natural antibiotic; protects against infection.
Selenium	Take 100 mcg daily.	As an antioxidant, it helps protect the body from infections.
Vitamin C	Take 1500 mg daily.	Speeds up healing and is an antioxidant.
Vitamin E	Take 400 IU daily.	An antioxidant that aids oxygen uptake by cells and enhances antibody production.

HOMEOPATHIC TREATMENT

Dissolve the tablets under your tongue. Do not eat or drink for fifteen minutes prior to or after taking medication. (See Part One, Homeopathy, for additional information.)

107

Preparation	Directions for Use	Comments
Belladonna 30X	Take 1 tablet hourly as needed.	Indicated for relief of fever and pain.
Hepar sulphuris 6X	Take 1 tablet 3 times a day.	To speed healing when infection is accompanied by pus.
Mercurius cyanatus 3X	Take 1 tablet 3 times a day.	Helps relieve pain and swelling of salivary glands.

HERBAL TREATMENT

Herb	Directions for Use	Comments
Hops	Prepare as tea (see Part Three, Using Herbs, Tea Preparation). Drink 2–3 cups daily, or take tablets as directed on package.	Helps improve circulation; good for stress and pain.
Licorice root	Prepare as tea (see Part Three, Using Herbs, Tea Preparation). Drink 2–3 cups daily.	High in vitamin B complex. Beneficial for stress control; helps reduce inflammation; promotes healthy immune system.
Sarsaparilla	Prepare as tea (see Part Three, Using Herbs, Tea Preparation). Drink 2–3 cups daily, or take tablets as directed on package.	Reduces fever.

RECOMMENDATIONS

■ Yogurt or acidophilus should be taken daily to help detoxify the system and balance the microorganisms in the body.

■ Drink plenty of fluids, especially water and grape juice. Grape juice is known for its blood-purifying properties.

■ A properly functioning immune system is the best defense against infections. Good nutrition, fresh air, exercise, and management of stress contribute to a healthy immune system.

■ It is important for expectant mothers to prevent infection, especially during the first three and last three months of pregnancy. Serious birth defects and damage to developing teeth may result from infections during this time.

■ *See also* Abscess; Gum Disease; Oral Herpes Infections; Yeast Infection, Oral, in Part Two.

Jaw Fracture

The jaw can be broken due to a severe blow to the face as in an accident, or it can be fractured intentionally to reset the bones for cosmetic reasons or to correct an improper previous setting. The simplest fracture to treat is one involving the bone, and not the skin or other tissues. When the fracture involves the skin and tissues inside the mouth, it becomes more complicated since any wounds in the skin can result in an infection.

Signs of a fractured jaw include great pain upon movement, a protruding bone on either the upper or lower jaw, or a change in the position of the teeth so they do not meet as they used to. Seek treatment immediately from a hospital or oral surgeon. If help is not immediately available, apply a temporary head bandage until you can get professional treatment (see figure in the margin). Wrap one bandage under the chin and tie it on top of the head. Wrap another bandage around the forehead. Be sure to loosen the bandage if it becomes too tight.

CONVENTIONAL TREATMENT

After a fracture, the jaw is placed in its proper position, and then it is immobilized by means of wiring, pins, and splints. The sooner an oral surgeon or maxillofacial specialist sets the jaw, the easier it is to regain correct positioning.

NUTRITIONAL SUPPLEMENTS

Supplement	Directions for Use	Comments
Calcium	Take 1500 mg daily.	Important component of bone and muscles; aids in bone calcification.
Magnesium	Take 750 mg daily.	Works in conjunction with calcium as a constituent of bone.
Vitamin B$_3$ (niacin)	Take 100 mg daily.	Alleviates muscle weakness and helps to heal injury.
Vitamin C	Take 2000 mg daily.	Enhances wound healing and repair of connective tissue.

HOMEOPATHIC TREATMENT

Dissolve the tablets under your tongue. Do not eat or drink for fifteen minutes prior to or after taking medication. (See Part One, Homeopathy, for additional information.)

Preparation	Directions for Use	Comments
Arnica 30X	Take 1 tablet hourly.	Improves healing of muscle and bone after injury.
Calcarea carbonica 6X	Take 1 tablet 2 times weekly.	Alleviates severe pain.
Hypericum 6X	Take 1 tablet 2 times daily.	Heals damaged nerves after trauma or injury.
Rhus toxicodendron 30X	Take 1 tablet 3 times daily.	Promotes healing of jaw joint.
Ruta 6X	Take 1 tablet 3 times daily.	Helps relieve pain and promotes union of bone.

FIRST AID

✚ After an accident or other trauma, if you find that you cannot move your jaw and there is severe pain, try to keep your jaw still and seek help immediately. If medical care is not immediately available, wrap a bandage around your head as shown in figure below.

✚ Apply ice to the outside area immediately.

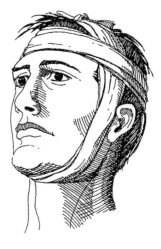

Temporary Head Bandage
For a fractured jaw, use a temporary head bandage until you can get medical help. Wrap one bandage under your chin and tie it on top of your head. Wrap a second bandage around your forehead.

HERBAL TREATMENT

Herb	Directions for Use	Comments
Chamomile	Prepare as a poultice (see Part Three, Using Herbs, Application Preparation).	Relieves pain and swelling.
Comfrey	Prepare as a poultice (see Part Three, Using Herbs, Application Preparation).	Helpful for healing of bruises.
Skullcap, chamomile, and lobelia	Prepare together or separately as tea (see Part Three, Using Herbs, Tea Preparation). Drink as needed.	Promotes relaxation.

RECOMMENDATIONS

■ To help reduce swelling and relieve pain, apply ice to the outside area immediately after the fracture. The following day, apply moist heat to help relieve pain.

■ The less the jaw is moved, the better it will set.

■ Once a fractured jaw is set, a liquid or soft-food diet is a must, depending on the extent of the wiring. The diet should be nutritious and balanced, containing mostly vegetables and fruits.

■ *See also* Diet and Nutrition in Part One.

Knocked-Out Tooth

See Tooth, Loss of; Trauma to Children's Teeth.

Lip- and Cheek-Biting

FIRST AID

✚ If you bite your lip or cheek hard enough, you may cause it to bleed. To stop the bleeding, press clean gauze and ice firmly against the area.

Many people habitually bite or suck their upper or lower lips. Although this habit can occur at any age, it is most common among children. Constant sucking or biting of the lips scrapes off any oil, leaving the lips extremely dry, crusty, and chapped. Typically, a child with this habit will have a red ring around the mouth. Usually, the lip that is most sucked or bitten will swell.

As a result of constantly biting or sucking the lower lip, the upper front teeth may not make contact with the lower; there will be a space between them. Biting or sucking the top lip can cause the top front teeth to be pushed in; if the condition is severe enough, orthodontic treatment may be required.

With cheek-biting, a line or clusters of small, red, slightly swollen spots are noticeable on the inside surface of the cheek. If this is a long-term habit, one or both cheeks may have a sucked-in appearance.

CONVENTIONAL TREATMENT

The dentist will advise the parent if orthodontic treatment is needed as a result of lip-biting or sucking. Moisturizers, balms, and ointments may be suggested to soothe the area, and the importance of stopping the habit should be discussed.

   Although cheek-biting does not cause damage to the teeth, it will cause the inside of the cheeks to become sore and irritated. The best treatment is to stop the habit. Sometimes cheek-biting may be due to improperly placed crowns or dentures. If this is the case, the dentist must correct the bite.

NUTRITIONAL SUPPLEMENTS

Supplement	Directions for Use	Comments
Multivitamin	Children should take a multi-vitamin according to the physician's directions.	Promotes healing.
Vitamin B_1	Take 100 mg daily.	Suggested for sensitivity of the inner lining of the cheeks.
Vitamin B_6	Take 100 mg daily.	Helps heal cracks, itching, and scaling around the mouth.
Vitamin B_{12}	Take 3 mcg daily.	Indicated for healing of sores in the inner lining of the cheeks.
Vitamin B complex	Take 100 mg daily.	May be substituted for the above B vitamins with the same benefits.
Vitamin C	Take 1500 mg daily.	Promotes healing.

HOMEOPATHIC TREATMENT

Dissolve the tablets under your tongue. Do not eat or drink for fifteen minutes prior to or after taking medication. (See Part One, Homeopathy, for additional information.)

Preparation	Directions for Use	Comments
Aconite 30X	Take 1 tablet 3 times daily.	Reduces anxiety, nervousness, restlessness.
Ambra grisia 3X	Take 1 tablet daily.	Reduces nervousness in children.
Antimonium crudum 6X	Take 1 tablet daily.	Helps heal and soothe dry, cracked lips.

HERBAL TREATMENT

Herb	Directions for Use	Comments
Anise	Prepare as a mouthwash (see Part Three, Using Herbs, Mouthwash Preparation). Use as needed.	Relieves sore, inflamed lips.

Catnip	Prepare as a tea (see Part Three, Using Herbs, Tea Preparation) and drink 1 cup in the morning and another at bedtime. Or take 500-mg capsule daily.	Calms the nervous system and soothes the irritability that may be contributing to lip- and cheek-biting.
Skullcap	Prepare as a tea (see Part Three, Using Herbs, Tea Preparation) and drink 1 cup in the morning and another at bedtime. Or take 500-mg capsule daily.	Calms the nervous system and soothes the irritability that may be contributing to lip- and cheek-biting.
Wood betony	Prepare as a tea (see Part Three, Using Herbs, Tea Preparation) and drink 1 cup in the morning and another at bedtime. Or take 500-mg capsule daily.	Calms the nervous system and soothes the irritability that may be contributing to lip- and cheek-biting.

RECOMMENDATIONS

■ Every time the lip- or cheek-biting habit is noticed, a gentle reminder to the child— especially a young child—will help eliminate the harmful pattern.

■ While working on breaking the habit, temporarily chewing sugarless gum may be helpful.

■ *See also* Orthodontic Techniques in Part Three.

Lips, Cracked

Cracked lips are common and may be caused by riboflavin deficiency, overexposure to the sun, ill-fitting dentures, lip-biting, or lip-sucking. Once cracks begin, there is a tendency to lick the lips, which causes the lips to dehydrate, making the condition worse. When the lips are licked, they are temporarily wet with saliva, which evaporates, causing drying. Furthermore, saliva contains digestive enzymes, which are not very moisturizing. As cracked lips worsen, they may bleed and there may be a burning sensation.

Ultraviolet rays from the sun are as damaging to the lips as they are to the rest of the skin. Sun damage to the lips causes dryness and cracks. Dry, cracked lips, especially at the corners of the mouth, is also a sign of riboflavin deficiency. Ill-fitting dentures can also lead to cracked lips. If the upper and lower teeth are not set properly in relationship to each other, or if teeth are lost or worn, a reduction in the vertical dimension of the bite results. With this condition, the lips overlap more, and creasing at the corners of the lips occurs. Saliva then seeps into the creases, causing cracks.

CONVENTIONAL TREATMENT

Some form of lip balm such as petroleum jelly is recommended for cracked lips. However, determining and eliminating the cause are essential factors in treatment.

Ill-fitting dentures should be corrected. Riboflavin supplements may be required to correct deficiencies. When exposed to sun and wind, be sure to use a lip balm containing sun block.

NUTRITIONAL SUPPLEMENTS

Supplement	Directions for Use	Comments
Vitamin B$_2$ (riboflavin)	Take 100 mg daily.	Will help eliminate cracked lips if they are due to riboflavin deficiency.
Vitamin E	Take 400 IU daily. Rub oil on lips.	Relieves dry, cracked lips.

HOMEOPATHIC TREATMENT

Dissolve the tablets under your tongue. Do not eat or drink for fifteen minutes prior to or after taking medication. (See Part One, Homeopathy, for additional information.)

Preparation	Directions for Use	Comments
Antimonium crudum 6X	Take 1 tablet 3 times daily.	Relieves dry lips and cracks at corner of mouth.
Arum triphyllum 30X	Take 1 tablet daily.	Protects and heals lips that are chapped and cracked with a burning sensation.
Natrum muriaticum 30X	Take 1 tablet daily.	Relieves dry lips and cracks at corner of mouth.

HERBAL TREATMENT

Herb	Directions for Use	Comments
Aloe vera	Place gel on a cotton-tipped swab (see Part Three, Using Herbs, Application Preparation). Apply directly to lips.	Helps heal burning, cracked, chapped lips.

RECOMMENDATIONS

■ Always use a sun block when outdoors.

■ To prevent dehydration, always drink plenty of water.

■ Avoid toothpastes with harsh chemicals that may irritate the lips or cause allergic reactions.

■ Apply ointment containing zinc oxide to protect the lips against bacteria or fungal infections seeping into cracks.

■ Avoid constant biting of the lips, as it will eventually cause dry, cracked lips.

■ *See also* Lip- and Cheek-Biting in Part Two.

Loss of Filling

See First Aid in Part Three.

Loss of Tooth

See Tooth, Loss of.

Malocclusion

See Orthodontic Problems.

Mercury Toxicity

The fillings referred to as "silver" are actually a mixture of silver, tin, copper, and mercury, and are more properly called amalgam fillings. The silver, tin, and copper are provided in a powder form by various manufacturers, with silver being the major constituent (40 to 70 percent), and tin and copper constituting 4 to 33 percent each, depending on the manufacturer. This powder is then mixed rapidly with mercury in a special machine, usually by the dental assistant, yielding a liquid that is from 50 to 60 percent mercury. The filling material is then placed in the tooth and smoothed with various dental tools.

Since the 1970s, there has been controversy in the dental profession regarding the safety of mercury as a filling material. Some dentists contend that no matter what the amount used in dental fillings, the mercury is toxic. At the same time, the American Dental Association (ADA) asserts that only a small percentage of individuals exhibit allergies to mercury, and that once mercury is mixed and hardened as a filling material, the percentage of individuals who are sensitive to it becomes even smaller.

While the ADA has maintained that mercury in amalgam is stable, various researchers have demonstrated that it is not. In 1970, dentist Wallace Johnson and others published the results of their research in *Journal of the American Dental Association*. The report indicated that "mercury, an essential element of dental amalgams, is not a stable material but one that vaporizes at ordinary temperatures." In 1985, the *Journal of Dental Research* published a report by dentists Murry Vimy and F.L. Lorscheider, who also claimed that mercury vapor is released from amalgam fillings. These researchers further stated that the vapor is then distributed throughout the body via the respiratory system, but accumulates mostly in the brain, kidneys, and gastrointestinal tract. Some of the symptoms associated with mercury toxicity include a metallic taste in the mouth, severe headaches, dizziness, fatigue, weakness, depression, hair loss, memory loss, coma, and death. Furthermore, a natural balance of microorganisms in the body is upset by excess mercury in the gastrointestinal tract, and this imbalance may lead to candida.

In addition, the previously mentioned researchers have reported that when the metal comes in contact with saliva, there is a "battery effect" in which currents are generated, causing mercury molecules from the surface of the fillings to be released into the tissues.

Another negative report was published in the *Journal of Prosthetic Dentistry* in 1983. David Eggleston, a dentist in private practice and a researcher and professor at the University of Southern California School of Dentistry, indicated that when amalgam and nickel-based fillings are present, there is a reduction in the T-lymphocytes of the immune system. Lymphocytes are white blood cells that are the core of the body's immune system. Lymphocytes that circulate through the thymus gland are called T-lymphocytes (thymocytes). They recognize foreign invaders in the body and form antibodies against them. Eggleston concluded that the introduction of mercury into the body might weaken the immune system by reducing the number of T-lymphocytes.

People are exposed to mercury not just through dental fillings, but also through certain foods, the air, pesticides, and sewage. However, fillings may be the largest single source of exposure to mercury. It is interesting to note that in Sweden, mercury amalgam fillings are banned.

If you presently have mercury fillings in your mouth, there is no need to panic and remove them. However, a few factors should be considered. As your amalgam fillings become old and require replacement, if you have no allergies to gold and cost is not a factor, gold is the best filling material. It is compatible with body tissues and can last up to twenty-five or thirty years. If the old fillings are too large and your dentist recommends a crown, one made of gold or porcelain with gold are equally acceptable. If cost is a factor, and you have no medical problems that can be traced to mercury sensitivity, then amalgam fillings may not be a negative health factor for you, and you can continue to have such fillings.

CONVENTIONAL TREATMENT

The ADA has set strict codes, which indicate that amalgam fillings may be replaced by composite or porcelain if the patient requests it for aesthetic reasons. However, there is a harsh penalty for the dentist who recommends removing fillings because of mercury toxicity.

Your dentist or medical doctor may order hair analysis if you suspect a problem. Although hair analysis indicates the presence of mercury levels in the body, it is not able to ascertain the actual source of the mercury contamination. Vapor analyzing machines such as the Jerome analyzer used by the National Air and Space Administration (NASA) can measure mercury vapor from fillings; however, such machines are not readily available.

Blood and urine are not reliable indicators of mercury toxicity, since mercury accumulates in tissues. However, dentist Hal Huggins, author of *It's All in Your*

DID YOU KNOW . . .
Mercury (Hg), sometimes known as quicksilver, is named for the speedy Roman god who served as messenger for the other gods. The silver-white chemical is the only common metal that is a liquid at room temperature. It is used in thermometers, barometers, and some batteries, as well as in dental amalgams.

Head, recommends a blood serum profile. He has found that when the body is affected by high levels of toxic mercury, the blood serum profile will indicate high glucose, low cholesterol, and slightly elevated globulin levels. He has also found that mercury interferes with the production of coenzyme A, which is necessary for the formation of hemoglobin. Huggins also recommends a urinary mercury excretion test. He maintains that porphyrins, chemicals manufactured by the body for the transporting of energy, are excreted in excessive amounts in the presence of high mercury levels. Some dentists use an electrical meter called an ammeter, which charts the positive and negative currents being generated from fillings. It is assumed that high negative currents (more than 4 microamps of current) may contain mercury molecules.

NUTRITIONAL SUPPLEMENTS

Supplement	Directions for Use	Comments
Beta-carotene	Take 15,000 IU daily.	Works as a scavenger of free radicals.
Garlic	Take two 250-mg tablets 3 times a day.	Helps strengthen the immune system.
Selenium	Take 200 mcg daily.	Helps detoxify heavy metals in the body.
Vitamin A	Take 25,000 IU daily.	As an antioxidant, protects cells from free radicals.
Vitamin B complex	Take 100 mg daily.	Helps to improve function of the central nervous system.
Vitamin C	Take 2000 mg daily beginning one week before removal of amalgam fillings.	Works as a scavenger to help remove toxic metals from tissues in the body.
Vitamin E	Take 400 IU daily.	Detoxifies the system and augments the action of selenium.

HOMEOPATHIC TREATMENT

Dissolve the tablets under your tongue. Do not eat or drink for fifteen minutes prior to or after taking medication. (See Part One, Homeopathy, for additional information.)

Preparation	Directions for Use	Comments
Hypericum 30X	Take 1 tablet hourly after a deep cavity has been filled.	Relieves pain and prevents nerve trauma.
Mercurius solubilis 30X	Take 1 tablet 3 times daily.	Helps eliminate toxic effects of mercury.
Mercurius vivus 30X	Beginning 1 week before removal of amalgam filling, take 1 tablet 3 times daily. Continue for 1 week following removal of filling.	Helps eliminate toxic effects of mercury.

HERBAL TREATMENT

Herb	Directions for Use	Comments
Alfalfa	Prepare as tea (see Part Three, Using Herbs, Tea Preparation). Drink 2–3 cups daily or take tablets as directed on package.	An excellent blood purifier and a good source of trace minerals.
Gentian	Prepare as tea (see Part Three, Using Herbs, Tea Preparation). Drink 2–3 cups daily or take tablets as directed on package.	A good blood purifier; helps strengthen the digestive system.

RECOMMENDATIONS

■ Chelation therapy is useful if you suspect mercury toxicity. (See Chelation Therapy in Part Three.)

■ As your present amalgam fillings become old and need to be replaced, consider using a different kind of filling material.

■ When removing old amalgam fillings or when placing them, it may be advisable for the dentist to use a dental dam. This square rubber sheet is placed and secured around the mouth and throat, exposing only the tooth or teeth to be worked on. This prevents particles of old fillings from going down the throat or becoming lodged in the gum tissues. Dental dams may be used for any procedure, but because they are time-consuming to put in place, many dentists do not use them.

■ It has been shown that as old amalgam fillings are removed, a high concentration of mercury vapor is produced in the area around the patient's mouth. To minimize the vapor, water spray should be used during the drilling along with high speed suction to collect most of the material.

■ It may be safer to remove one amalgam filling at a time due to the increased amount of mercury vapor given off during replacement.

■ When old amalgam fillings are replaced, drink eight ounces of distilled water mixed with two teaspoons of cider vinegar and honey to taste. This is an excellent detoxifier that can be taken daily.

■ Dentist Hal Huggins has set up a protocol that uses a person's blood for testing the biocompatibility of dental materials and the person's immune system. This protocol is described in detail in his book, *It's All in Your Head* (Avery Publishing Group, Garden City Park, NY).

Migraine Headache

A throbbing migraine headache usually occurs on one side of the head or behind one eye, and is often accompanied by nausea, vomiting, blurred vision, and tingling and numbness in the limbs that can last for a few hours or days. A classic migraine is preceded by sensations called auras, which can consist of sensory disturbances, speech disorders, and general weakness. Visual disturbances can consist of brilliant stars, sparks, flashes, or simple geometric forms that pass across the visual field. Other disturbances include tingling sensations, dizziness, ringing in the ears, or feeling that a part of the body is distorted in size or shape.

Widening blood vessels, which result in spasms, are directly related to the head pain. The exact cause of migraines is not known, although allergic reactions, constipation, stress, excess carbohydrates, iodine-rich foods, alcohol, loud noises, and bright lights can bring on attacks. Temporomandibular joint syndrome (TMJ)—an abnormal condition of the muscles and joints connecting the upper and lower jaw—is another possible trigger of migraine headaches. For further information, see TMJ in Part Two.

Mouth-Breathing-Related Problems

Mouth-breathing is usually caused by blocked nasal passages or a gap (anterior open bite) between the upper front teeth and the lower front teeth. Mouth-breathing produces a dry mouth—a dehydrated environment in which bacteria can thrive and cause cavities. Mouth-breathers are also more likely to snore and to have bad breath and dry, cracked lips.

CONVENTIONAL TREATMENT

Correcting the cause of mouth-breathing is the treatment of choice. Surgery may be needed to correct the blockage in the nasal passages. Thumb-sucking and tongue-thrusting, which are some of the causes of an anterior open bite, should be intercepted at an early age before damage is done.

NUTRITIONAL SUPPLEMENTS

Supplement	Directions for Use	Comments
Coenzyme Q-10	Take 30 mg daily.	Improves circulation by enhancing oxygen uptake by tissues in the mouth.
Vitamin B complex	Take 100 mg daily.	Combats anxiety and stress.
Vitamin C	Take 1500 mg daily.	Prevents sore gums.

HOMEOPATHIC TREATMENT

Dissolve the tablets under your tongue. Do not eat or drink for fifteen minutes prior to or after taking medication. (See Part One, Homeopathy, for additional information.)

118

Preparation	Directions for Use	Comments
Bryonia 6X	Take 1 tablet 3 times daily.	For relief of dry mouth, tongue, and throat.
Lycopodium 6X	Take 1 tablet 3 times a week.	Use when dry mouth is accompanied by bad breath.
Nux moschata 6X	Take 1 tablet 3 times daily.	Indicated for extremely dry mouth and throat.

HERBAL TREATMENT

Herb	Directions for Use	Comments
Aloe vera	Place gel on a cotton-tipped swab (see Part Three, Using Herbs, Application Preparation). Rub on gums at bedtime.	Keeps moisture in tissues, preventing dehydration.
Dandelion	Prepare as tea (see Part Three, Using Herbs, Tea Preparation). Drink 2–3 cups daily, or take in tablet form as directed on package.	Effective as a blood purifier.
Gentian	Prepare as tea (see Part Three, Using Herbs, Tea Preparation). Drink 2–3 cups daily, or take in tablet form as directed on package.	Effective as a blood purifier.
Red clover	Prepare as tea (see Part Three, Using Herbs, Tea Preparation). Drink 2–3 cups daily, or take in tablet form as directed on package.	Effective as a blood purifier.
Rosemary	Prepare as a mouthwash (see Part Three, Using Herbs, Mouthwash Preparation). Rinse once in the morning and once at night.	Useful for bad breath, dry mouth, and dry throat.

RECOMMENDATIONS

■ Because people do not breathe through their mouths unless there is a problem with bite or nasal passages, the only way to eliminate mouth-breathing is to identify the cause and treat it.

■ Drink plenty of water (at least eight 8-ounce glasses per day), especially at bedtime. Melting ice cubes in the mouth may also help with dry mouth.

■ Discontinue all caffeinated beverages, including coffee, tea, hot chocolate, and cola drinks. In some individuals, caffeine has been reported to heighten anxiety and create nervousness, which commonly results in dry mouth.

■ Practice proper oral hygiene.

■ To help relieve dry mouth, rinses such as Xero-Lube or Salivart may be recommended. Biotene toothpaste may also be helpful.

■ *See also* Dry Mouth; Lip- and Cheek-Biting; Thumb-Sucking-Related Problems in Part Two.

119

Myofascial Pain Dysfunction (MPD)

See TMJ.

Nail-Biting

See Finger-Biting-Related Dental Problems.

Object Stuck Between Teeth

We all know how embarrassing and uncomfortable it is to have food or some other material stuck between our teeth. Too many of us, however, don't realize how harmful it can be to stick hard objects into the mouth in an attempt to dislodge the offending object.

To safely loosen something stuck between your teeth, first try rinsing vigorously with tepid water. If that doesn't work, use a balsa-wood wedge toothpick that you have first moistened in your mouth. Press the toothpick firmly against the side of the tooth, and move it in and out between the teeth, being careful not to bruise the gums. Repeat the rinsing and toothpick procedures as needed.

Flossing is another effective method for removing food particles or other objects that are trapped between teeth. For information on proper flossing technique, see Oral Hygiene, Flossing, in Part Three.

If, after a few attempts, you have been unsuccessful in removing the object, have your dentist remove it. This will prevent you from causing any damage to a tooth or tender gum tissue.

Oral Cancer

Oral cancer accounts for about 4 percent of all cancers. Occurring in all ethnic groups, it tends to first appear at age sixty or older. Men are twice as likely to be victims as women. Those who use tobacco and alcohol are at increased risk of oral cancer. Furthermore, spread of cancer from the mouth to the head and neck (about

20 percent of all cases) may be prevented if the use of tobacco and alcohol is terminated.

Although oral cancer may occur in any area of the mouth, the tongue is the most common site. The lip is the site of oral cancer in about 38 percent of all cases. Pipe- and cigarette-smoking, as well as overexposure to the sun, have all been implicated as causes of cancer of the lip. The third most common site is the floor of the mouth, under the tongue.

No reliable signs and symptoms are associated with oral cancer. However, the most common detectable sign is a painful ulcer. When a mouth tumor becomes malignant, it may appear as a white and/or red patch that is not painful. Since no pain is felt, most individuals delay seeking professional advice. As a result of this delay in treatment, the survival rate for victims of oral cancers averages less than 50 percent. At the advanced stage, the cancer commonly spreads to the neck, and, in about 15 percent of all cases, to other organs.

CONVENTIONAL TREATMENT

Once oral cancer is detected, radiation therapy and surgery are recommended. These forms of treatment are usually used in combination. Surgical techniques include the use of lasers, which are able to dissolve tumors by applying intense heat to a very confined area. Cryosurgery is a technique in which subfreezing temperatures are used to destroy cancerous tissue. Radiation dosage should not exceed 6500 rads, or it may have dangerous side effects on the tissues exposed to the radiation. As the cancer advances, chemotherapy is utilized. Currently, varying dosages and combinations of methotrexate, bleomycin, and cisplatin are used.

Once the above treatments have been administered, there may be side effects that must be addressed. For example, surgery may cause defects that can be corrected with maxillofacial prosthetic appliances. Radiation therapy frequently causes alterations in taste and saliva, interfering with diet and leading to the formation of numerous cavities. High levels of radiation destroy tooth tissue, another cause of cavities. Radiation therapy may lead to osteomyletis in the jaw—a serious form of infection that can be treated with antibiotics. And chemotherapy may cause loss of hair as well as other side effects, such as ulcers and bleeding gums, depending on the drugs used.

NUTRITIONAL SUPPLEMENTS

Supplement	Directions for Use	Comments
Beta-carotene	Take 10,000 IU daily.	Functions as an antioxidant, destroying free radicals.
Garlic	Take two 250-mg tablets 3 times daily.	Natural antibiotic; enhances immune system.
Kelp	Take five 500-mg tablets daily.	Excellent source of trace minerals.
Selenium	Take 100 mcg daily.	As an antioxidant, it acts as a scavenger of harmful elements in tissues.
Vitamin A	Take 25,000 IU daily.	Helps enhance immunity and is needed for maintenance of healthy tissue.
Vitamin C + bioflavonoids	Take 4000 mg daily.	Encourages and promotes repair of tissue.

Vitamin E	Take 400 IU daily.	As an antioxidant, it helps repair tissues and reduce scarring.
Zinc	Take 100 mg daily.	Improves sense of taste.

HOMEOPATHIC TREATMENT

When using tablets, dissolve them under your tongue. When using liquids, place the drops directly on your tongue. (Because of their alcohol base, liquids should not be used by children or recovering alcoholics.) Do not eat or drink for fifteen minutes prior to or after taking medication. (See Part One, Homeopathy, for additional information.)

Preparation	Directions for Use	Comments
Echinacea rudbeckia 6X	Take 5–10 drops every 2 hours.	Indicated for dry swollen tongue, dry mouth, sores and cracks on lips and tongue, and gums that bleed easily. Promotes the flow of saliva.
Formalin 3X	Take 1 tablet daily.	Helps restore lost sense of taste.
Hepar sulphuris 30X	Take 1 tablet 3 times daily.	Promotes healing of infection and painful, bleeding gums. Relieves depression and anxiety.
Mercurius solubilis 6X	Take 1 tablet 3 times daily.	Indicated for healing of swollen glands, infections, and ulcers.
Phytolacca 30X	Take 5 drops hourly.	Indicated for swollen glands, and for difficulty when swallowing.

HERBAL TREATMENT

Herb	Directions for Use	Comments
Alfalfa	Prepare as a tea (see Part Three, Using Herbs, Tea Preparation). Drink as often as possible.	Excellent blood purifier.
Aloe vera	Place gel on cotton-tipped swab (see Part Three, Using Herbs, Application Preparation). Apply directly on sores. Do not eat or drink for at least 1 hour after applying gel.	Very soothing for mouth sores.
Chickweed	Prepare as a mouthwash (see Part Three, Using Herbs, Mouthwash Preparation). Rinse every night or 3 times a week.	Relieves irritated, dry mouth.
Dandelion root	Prepare as a tea (see Part Three, Using Herbs, Tea Preparation). Drink as often as possible.	Excellent blood purifier.

Goldenseal	Prepare as a mouthwash (see Part Three, Using Herbs, Mouthwash Preparation). Rinse nightly. Prepare as an application (see Part Three, Using Herbs, Application Preparation) and apply to your lips as needed for relief.	Relieves sores and ulcers in the mouth and on the lips.
Red clover	Prepare as a tea (see Part Three, Using Herbs, Tea Preparation). Drink 2–3 cups daily.	Excellent blood purifier.
Rockrose	Prepare as a tea (see Part Three, Using Herbs, Tea Preparation). Drink ¼ cup daily. Prepare as a mouthwash (see Part Three, Using Herbs, Mouthwash Preparation) and use as needed.	Relieves mouth sores.
Violet	Prepare as a mouthwash (see Part Three, Using Herbs, Mouthwash Preparation). Rinse morning and night.	Effective for healing ulcers.

RECOMMENDATIONS

■ To prevent dry mouth during radiation therapy, sugarless candy drops or gum, may be helpful.

■ Cavities formed as a result of radiation exposure should be filled as soon as possible.

■ Cancer therapy tends to cause fewer dental problems for those with clean mouths. Proper home oral hygiene is, therefore, extremely important, as are professional cleanings.

■ Commercial mouthwashes are not recommended since they contain chemicals that may be absorbed by the tissues in the mouth, indirectly affecting the healing process of the mouth sores.

■ Biotene toothpaste, mouthwash, and chewing gum are specially formulated for dry mouth. Grace toothpaste with aloe vera and vitamin C is also recommended.

■ The importance of a balanced, nutritious diet cannot be stressed enough. Drink plenty of water and eat fresh fruits and vegetables. It may be preferable to obtain organically grown fruits and vegetables; these do not contain pesticides.

■ Some researchers are finding that shark cartilage is helpful in treating certain cancers, including some oral cancers. Information about the research can be found in Dr. I. William Lane's book *Sharks Don't Get Cancer* (Avery Publishing, Garden City Park, NY).

■ State of mind is also extremely important in how well the body responds to treatment. Tension, anxiety, fear, and worry will deplete energy, place an extra burden on the immune system, and rob the body of vital nutrients. Try to maintain a positive attitude.

■ *See also* Cysts and Tumors in Part Two.

Oral Herpes Infections

Herpes viruses are a group of viruses that cause painful skin eruptions. This entry involves those forms of the herpes virus that cause oral problems. The herpes simplex virus (HSV1), which involves the mouth area, includes primary herpes (herpetic stomatitis) and recurrent herpes simplex. The herpes varicella-zoster virus is another form of herpes that may affect the mouth.

Primary herpes is a common virus and usually appears in infants and children. It is frequently present with pneumonia, meningitis, and upper respiratory infections. Clusters of small blisterlike elevations (vesicles), the size of a pinhead to a split pea, may appear throughout the gums, inner lining of the lips and cheeks, roof of the mouth, tongue, and throat. Along with pain, symptoms include high fever, headache, loss of appetite, swollen lymph glands, increased salivation, foul breath, and a general feeling of discomfort. In infants and young children, this form of herpes can be dangerous because of the problems of dehydration, high fever (as high as 105°F), and spread of infection to the hands and eyes through hand contact. The virus usually runs its course within fourteen days without scar formation. Many infected people continue to harbor the virus in nerve fibers and may experience recurrent attacks.

The most common adult form of herpes virus is the recurrent herpes simplex, in which small blisterlike elevations appear on the lips, gums, and palate. Usually, these elevations are triggered by upper respiratory infection or fever, which is why they are commonly called fever blisters or cold sores. Herpes simplex is also commonly triggered by too much exposure to sun, by trauma, or by an immune system weakened by various illnesses. Symptoms include tingling or itching, which lasts for a few hours, and pain, which may last one to two days. The vesicles then appear and are often very painful. Within forty-eight hours, the vesicles form ulcers and then scabs. Healing is usually complete within eight to ten days.

Like HSV1, herpes varicella-zoster infections have a primary and recurrent form. The primary form is typically associated with chickenpox. Mouth ulcers, fever, discomfort, swollen glands, and a rash on the trunk of the body and face are some of the symptoms. This form of herpes usually heals within seven to fourteen days. The recurrent form of herpes zoster, also called shingles, affects adults and usually spreads along a nerve path. If the virus affects a nerve in the head or face, there is frequently pain along the infected nerve accompanied by a rash and mouth ulcers. If the nerves inside the mouth are infected, ulcers will be present on the tongue and gums, and the teeth may even be painful.

There are other forms of the herpes virus that do not involve the mouth area. These include herpes simplex virus 2 (HSV2), which involves the genitals; zoster oticus, which affects the facial nerves; and the Epstein-Barr virus, which causes mononucleosis.

CONVENTIONAL TREATMENT

There is no known cure for any of the herpes infections. However, when fever and pain are present, Tylenol, aspirin, or other analgesic is often recommended. Other medications that may be recommended include lidocaine ointment, which numbs the pain; Benadryl, which relieves allergic reactions and may act as a sedative;

gentian violet and methylene blue, which help numb the pain; and over-the-counter ointments such as Orabase, which gives temporary relief from the symptoms. If the infections are frequent and interfere with eating and other functions, an antiviral drug called acyclovir (Zovirax) may be prescribed.

NUTRITIONAL SUPPLEMENTS

Supplement	Directions for Use	Comments
Garlic	Take two 500-mg tablets, 3 times daily.	Strengthens immune system and acts as a natural antibiotic.
L-lysine	Take 500-mg tablets 2 times daily.	Stops pain and spread of infection. However, dosage must be maintained after sores have disappeared or they will recur.
Vitamin A + beta-carotene	Take 20,000 IU daily.	Promotes health of the inner lining of the mouth.
Vitamin B complex	Take 100 mg daily.	Improves transport of oxygen to cells; has an important function in metabolism and health of the nervous system. Helps decrease stress.
Vitamin B_{12}	Take 4 mcg daily.	Speeds healing of vesicles.
Vitamin C + bioflavonoids	Take 2000 mg daily.	Speeds healing of vesicles.

HOMEOPATHIC TREATMENT

Dissolve the tablets under your tongue. Do not eat or drink for fifteen minutes prior to or after taking medication. (See Part One, Homeopathy, for additional information.)

Preparation	Directions for Use	Comments
Capsicum 6X	Take 1 tablet 3 times daily as needed.	Promotes relief of mouth odor, pain, and vesicles.
Mercurius solubilis 30X	Take 1 tablet 3 times daily as needed.	Helps relieve pain from mouth sores.
Natrum muriaticum 30X	Take 1 tablet 3 times daily as needed.	Speeds healing of vesicles.
Rhus toxicodendron 30X	Take 1 tablet 3 times daily as needed.	Helps reduce swollen glands, fever blisters, and pain.

HERBAL TREATMENT

Herb	Directions for Use	Comments
Alfalfa	Prepare as a tea (see Part Three, Using Herbs, Tea Preparation). Drink 2–3 cups daily or take tablets as directed on package.	Excellent antioxidant and blood purifier.
Catnip	Prepare as a tea (see Part Three, Using Herbs, Tea Preparation). Drink 2 or more cups a day.	Indicated for calming the nervous system during times of stress.

| Rockrose | Prepare as a mouthwash (see Part Three, Using Herbs, Mouthwash Preparation) and rinse in the morning and at bedtime. | Useful for relief of painful herpes ulcers. |

RECOMMENDATIONS

■ Although Tylenol, aspirin, and other analgesics are commonly recommended for fever reduction, be aware that frequent use may result in serious side effects. Long-term use of acetaminophen (Tylenol) can be toxic to the liver, and excessive use of aspirin can cause intestinal bleeding. Aspirin has also been connected to Reye's syndrome in children.

■ If the mouth is so painful that you cannot eat or drink fluids, dehydration may result. If this is the case, consult with your physician.

■ A soft diet is preferred during an oral herpes outbreak, but if it is too difficult and painful to eat any foods, supplementation with vitamins and minerals is essential.

■ Corticosteroids and antibiotics are not advisable in any form. The use of corticosteroids is especially dangerous because it may result in a serious and possibly fatal spread of the infection.

■ Avoid caffeine, spicy foods, peanuts, chocolate, cashews, beer and other alcoholic beverages. These are rich in the amino acid L-arginine, on which the herpes virus thrives.

■ Avoid overexposure to sun and wind. Exercise and take steps to relieve stress. (Stress and lack of exercise weaken the body's defense mechanisms.)

Oral Tori

See Cysts and Tumors.

Orthodontic Problems

Orthodontic work may be required for any one of a number of reasons. If the jaw is too small to accommodate all of the teeth, certain teeth may be extracted to make room. Appliances—fixed or removable—are then placed to correct rotation of teeth. Appliances are also used to correct crossbite, a condition in which the lower teeth protrude over the upper. These appliances are sometimes necessary if baby teeth are lost too soon or too late, which can interfere with the normal positioning of permanent teeth. More severe imbalances are corrected with braces as well as a "head gear," which is used to reposition the jaw. In some instances, surgery is the only means by which the position of the jaw can be corrected.

Orthodontic problems are often caused by habits such as nail- and finger- biting, lip-biting, and thumb-sucking, which put constant pressure on the teeth.

See also Finger-Biting-Related Dental Problems; Lip- and Cheek-Biting; Thumb-Sucking-Related Problems in Part Two; and Orthodontic Techniques in Part Three.

Pain, Facial, Head, Muscle, and Neck

See TMJ.

Pain, Tooth

See Broken, Cracked, or Chipped Teeth; Cavities; Pain and Anxiety; TMJ; Toothache in Part Two; and First Aid in Part Three.

Pain and Anxiety

Fear and anxiety keep hundreds of individuals from seeking needed dental treatment, which may turn minor dental problems into major ones. Fear is usually caused by a bad experience with dental treatment, or from hearing about another individual's bad experience.

Negative experiences that occur during childhood visits to the dentist are hard to forget. It is important to understand that a child has no control over treatment situations and is at the mercy of the practitioner. If you fear dental treatment due to a past negative experience, follow the guidelines given in Choosing a Dentist in Part One until you have found a dentist with whom you feel comfortable. Once you have found a dentist in whom you have confidence and with whom you can communicate, half the battle is won.

Once you have seen a dentist and have received a diagnosis, get a clear understanding of what the treatment will involve. If the treatment involves pain, be sure to establish the procedure for blocking that pain before beginning treatment. (See Anesthesia; Stress and Anxiety Management in Part Three.) It is important to note that it is much easier for the dentist to concentrate on the technical aspects of treatment if the patient is relaxed. A stressed and nervous person finds it difficult to sit still and keep his or her mouth open adequately. This patient will also experience more pain because the nervous system will translate *any* sensations into pain. Most dentists want to finish treatment on this type of person as soon as possible because it causes stress on the dentist, as well. In other words, the more relaxed you are, the better chances you have of receiving the best possible treatment.

CONVENTIONAL TREATMENT

During all office procedures, the dentist is responsible for using the appropriate anesthesia to block pain. Should you experience any pain after leaving the office, a number of over-the-counter and prescription medications can help. One option is acetaminophen, the active ingredient in Tylenol, Panadol, Anacin-3, Tempra, and other over-the-counter pain-relievers. Keep in mind, though, that in high doses or in combination with alcohol, these drugs can be toxic to the liver. Ibuprofen is an anti-inflammatory that is also used to relieve pain. It is found in Advil, Medipren, Motrin, Nuprin, Pediaprofen, and in prescription drugs. Codeine, available by prescription only, is a narcotic used when pain is not relieved by other medications.

Aspirin, once the most commonly used over-the-counter analgesic, can cause intestinal bleeding; its use has also been connected to Reye's syndrome in children. Aspirin should not be used by children or teenagers, by those with a history of internal bleeding, or when there is heavy bleeding from a wound.

NUTRITIONAL SUPPLEMENTS

Supplement	Directions for Use	Comments
Calcium	Take 1500 mg daily at bedtime.	Anxiety is sometimes related to low levels of calcium.
Magnesium	Take 750 mg daily.	Works with calcium to help relieve anxiety and insomnia.
Vitamin B complex	Take 100 mg daily.	Promotes a healthy nervous system, which is important in stress management.

HOMEOPATHIC TREATMENT

Dissolve the tablets under your tongue. Do not eat or drink for fifteen minutes prior to or after taking medication. (See Part One, Homeopathy, for additional information.)

Preparation	Directions for Use	Comments
Aconite 30X	Take 1 tablet 3 times a day on the day before treatment and on the day of treatment.	Useful for treatment of anxiety, nervousness, fear, physical and mental restlessness.
Ambra grisia 3X	Give children 1 tablet 3 times a day on the day before treatment and on the day of treatment.	Helpful for soothing nervousness.

| *Kali phosphoricum* 6X | Take 1 tablet 3 times a day on the day before treatment and 1 tablet hourly on the day of treatment. | Helps decrease worry and nervousness. |

HERBAL TREATMENT

Herb	Directions for Use	Comments
Catnip	Prepare as a tea (see Part Three, Using Herbs, Tea Preparation). Drink as needed.	Soothes nervous irritability.
Dill	Prepare as a tea (see Part Three, Using Herbs, Tea Preparation). Drink as needed.	Reduces nervousness.
Hops	Prepare as a tea (see Part Three, Using Herbs, Tea Preparation). Drink as needed.	Useful for restlessness and toothache.
Licorice root	Prepare as a tea (see Part Three, Using Herbs, Tea Preparation). Drink as needed.	Soothes nervous irritability.

RECOMMENDATIONS

■ Be patient with yourself; practice makes perfect. If you were not as relaxed in the dentist's chair as you had wanted, review whatever happened that caused your anxiety. Work on eliminating those causes.

■ You will notice that as you control your anxiety level, pain diminishes also.

■ Some dentists have found that having an anxious patient listen to music with headphones during a procedure promotes relaxation.

■ *See also* Stress and Anxiety Management in Part Three.

DID YOU KNOW . . .
Licorice, one of the most widely studied herbs, is an ancient Chinese medicinal. Its use dates back at least 4,000 years. Scientists have now confirmed that licorice exhibits several pharmacological actions. It has been shown to be anti-inflammatory and antibiotic, and effective in the treatment of ulcers. There is evidence that licorice's active ingredient (glycyrrhizin) inhibits the growth of plaque and is effective against *Streptococcus mutans*, the bacteria associated with cavity development. *Caution: Licorice should be avoided by those with high blood pressure, and by those taking digoxin-based drugs.*

Pericoronitis

See Wisdom-Teeth-Related Problems.

Periodontal Disease

See Gum Disease.

Periodontitis

See Gum Disease.

Plaque

Dental plaque is a high density population of microorganisms that adheres to the hard enamel surfaces of teeth. These bacteria use ingredients found in our diet and saliva along with products of their metabolism to grow. The presence of these microorganisms and their ability to grow and colonize on tooth surfaces can cause cavities and gum disease, which, left untreated, can destroy the teeth and their supporting structures.

Although streptococcal species constitute the largest percentage of bacteria in plaque, the microbial content of plaque is of a mixed population and is not static, but rather in a continuous state of change. For example, in the early stages of plaque development, certain bacterial strains are found; whereas, older more mature plaque contains other genera of bacteria. Samples of plaque may vary from tooth surface to tooth surface, and even from site to site on the same tooth surface.

Oral bacteria appear in the mouth of a newborn one week after birth. These first bacteria are *Streptococcus salivarius* and *Streptococcus mitis*, followed by *Veillonella* and a few other forms of bacteria that do not require oxygen to grow (anaerobic). After teeth erupt, a thin film composed primarily of salivary proteins becomes firmly attached to the surfaces of the teeth. This is followed by an increase in streptococcal species such as *Streptococcus mutans* and *Streptococcus sanguis*, both of which require hard tooth surfaces to colonize and grow. More bacteria follow, and by the time puberty is reached, the oral bacteria are that of an adult.

Carbohydrates and proteins become the energy sources used by bacteria to sustain life and growth. The amount, type, and frequency of carbohydrate consumption in our diets determine the types of bacteria present in plaque. For example, frequent intake of sucrose (ordinary granulated, powdered, or brown sugar; molasses; and maple syrup) enhances the colonization of *Streptococcus mutans*. Of all the sugars, sucrose is the most likely to promote dental plaque and bacterial growth because it is a source of fermentable energy for most of the microorganisms in plaque.

As the microorganisms in the plaque metabolize carbohydrates, they produce acids, particularly lactic acid, that dissolve the tooth surface. Recent studies comparing plaque samples taken from cavity-free teeth with samples taken from teeth with cavities show twice as much lactic acid on the cavity-ridden teeth. The more sucrose a person eats, the more harmful are the acids are found in plaque, and the more acidic the pH of the plaque. Nonetheless, the average American consumes an astounding 100 to 125 pounds of sugar per year.

The sugar substitutes available on the market today cannot be metabolized by the microorganisms in plaque. Xylitol has a sweetness rating similar to sucrose; however, the plaque microorganisms cannot metabolize it as readily. In a two-year study conducted in Turka, Finland, a 90-percent reduction in cavities was found in the group that used xylitol instead of sucrose. Xylitol is currently being used in many commercial food products and toothpastes, including Grace.

Aspartame (NutraSweet), another sweetening agent currently being used commercially, is approximately 200 times sweeter than sucrose; however, there is some concern that the phenylalanine and aspartate components of aspartame may be toxic. The carcinogenic potential of saccharin and sodium cyclamate, which are noncaloric synthetic sweeteners, has also been debated, and sugar alcohols such as mannitol and sorbitol produce gastrointestinal distress. In fact, sorbitol is often used as an active ingredient in laxatives.

CONVENTIONAL TREATMENT

A proper oral-hygiene regimen practiced at home, as well as routine professional cleanings are, of course, the most-often-recommended means of plaque control. Your dentist may also suggest that you have saliva tests to determine which type of bacteria are present in the greatest number. The dentist may then prescribe an antibiotic to destroy those bacteria.

NUTRITIONAL SUPPLEMENTS

Supplement	Directions for Use	Comments
Calcium	Take 1500 mg daily.	Important in maintaining healthy teeth and bones; prevents bone loss.
Coenzyme Q-10	Take 60 mg daily.	Improves circulation and uptake of oxygen to gums; promotes healing of gum disease.
Kelp	Take 500 mg daily.	Important source of trace minerals, needed for healthy teeth and bones.
Magnesium	Take 750 mg daily.	Works with calcium to enhance health of teeth and bones.
Phosphorus	Take 1500 mg daily.	Needed for bone and tooth formation; has been shown to help reduce cavity formation.
Vitamin C	Take 2000 mg daily.	Promotes healing of bleeding gums.

HOMEOPATHIC TREATMENT

Dissolve the tablets under your tongue. Do not eat or drink for fifteen minutes prior to or after taking medication. (See Part One, Homeopathy, for additional information.)

Preparation	Directions for Use	Comments
Mercurius solubilis 6X	Take 1 tablet daily.	Helps heal inflamed gums.
Staphysagria 30X	Take 1 tablet daily.	Helps heal gums that are bleeding and spongy.

HERBAL TREATMENT

Herb	Directions for Use	Comments
Alfalfa	Take 1000-mg tablet or capsule daily.	An excellent source of trace minerals and a blood purifier.
Goldenseal	Prepare as a mouthwash (see Part Three, Using Herbs, Mouthwash Preparation). Rinse as needed.	Helps heal gum disease.
Myrrh	Prepare as a mouthwash (see Part Three, Using Herbs, Mouthwash Preparation). Rinse as needed.	Helps heal gum disease.

RECOMMENDATIONS

■ Various mouthwashes and toothpastes claim to control plaque; however, the mechanical actions of daily brushing and flossing do more to accomplish this goal. (See Oral Hygiene in Part Three.)

■ Daily rinses with a baking soda solution (see Part Three, Using Herbs, Mouthwash Preparation) and use of a toothpaste containing baking soda are excellent ways to reduce the acid level in your mouth.

■ Diet is extremely important in preventing plaque build-up on teeth and gums. Reduce consumption of carbohydrates, and increase consumption of raw vegetables, whole grains, and fresh fruits.

■ Rough surfaces on teeth, at the edges of crowns and fillings, or underneath bridges; implants; and fillings increase the accumulation of plaque. If these areas are not cleaned properly, plaque build-up may cause tooth damage and/or gum disease.

■ For the health of your teeth, avoid sugar and use sugar substitutes if you must.

■ *See also* Hygiene Basics; Diet and Nutrition in Part One; and Oral Hygiene in Part Three.

Pyorrhea

See Gum Disease.

Receding Gums

See Gums, Receding.

Root Canal Therapy

Root canal therapy is designed to treat endodontic problems—those associated with the tooth root, dental pulp, and surrounding tissue, including blood vessels and nerves. Specifically, root canal therapy (endodontic therapy) involves any dental procedure that attempts to protect normal pulp tissue, as well as to medicate or actually remove diseased pulp tissue.

See also Endodontic Problems in Part Two; and Endodontic Techniques in Part Three.

Salivary Gland Disorders

Saliva is manufactured by three pairs of salivary glands—the parotid, sublingual, and submandibular—as shown in the margin figure. Disorders of the salivary glands affect the flow of saliva, causing dry mouth and impacting the mouth's general health.

Sialolithiasis is a collection of calcium compounds that forms in the salivary glands or ducts. If these stones block a duct, the flow of saliva is stopped. The obstruction causes pressure in the gland, making it swollen and painful.

Mumps, a viral infection, causes the parotid salivary glands to become swollen and painful. Benign and malignant tumors may also develop in the parotid glands—as well as in the other salivary glands—causing pain and swelling.

When one of the small salivary glands in the lining of the mouth is damaged due to trauma, trapped saliva forms a cyst resembling a blister. These mucus-retention cysts, or mucoceles, are usually seen on the lower lip and under the tongue in the floor of the mouth. When these cysts affect a major salivary gland, they are called ranula.

Cat-scratch disease, caused by the parasite *Bedsonia*, often affects the lymph nodes and/or the parotid salivary glands. Symptoms include swelling of the affected gland, pain, fever, chills, nausea, and headache. In most cases, the disease regresses within six weeks; however, it sometimes lasts as long as six months.

Sjogren's disease causes enlargement of the salivary glands; dry mouth, throat, and eyes; and arthritis. It is seen mostly in middle-aged and elderly women. Although its cause is not known, it is believed to be an autoimmune disease.

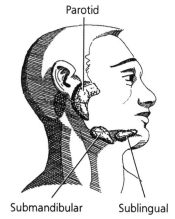

Parotid

Submandibular   Sublingual

Salivary Glands

133

CONVENTIONAL TREATMENT

Stones in the salivary glands are usually removed surgically, as are mucoceles. Malignant tumors are treated with radiation, surgery, and chemotherapy. Treatment for Sjogren's disease consists of hormonal, vitamin, or antibiotic therapy. Mumps are rarely seen today, as children are immunized against it.

NUTRITIONAL SUPPLEMENTS

Supplement	Directions for Use	Comments
Vitamin A + beta-carotene	Take 15,000 IU daily.	Aids and promotes proper functioning of the immune system.
Vitamin C	Take 2000 mg daily.	Important antioxidant; speeds the healing process.
Vitamin E	Take 400 IU daily.	Destroys free radicals and enhances the immune system.

HOMEOPATHIC TREATMENT

Dissolve the tablets under your tongue. Do not eat or drink for fifteen minutes prior to or after taking medication. (See Part One, Homeopathy, for additional information.)

Preparation	Directions for Use	Comments
Bryonia 6X	Take 1 tablet 2 times daily.	Helps gum tissues irritated by extreme dry mouth.
Pulsatilla 6X	Take 1 tablet 3 times daily.	Improves dry mouth accompanied by bad breath.

HERBAL TREATMENT

Herb	Directions for Use	Comments
Aloe vera	Place gel on a cotton-tipped swab (see Part Three, Using Herbs, Application Preparation) and rub on gums. Do not eat or drink for at least 1 hour after applying gel.	Helps soothe and heal irritated gums.
Eucalyptus oil	Place on a cotton-tipped swab and rub on gums.	Soothes irritated gums.
Goldenseal	Mix with baking soda and prepare as a mouthwash (see Part Three, Using Herbs, Mouthwash Preparation). Rinse in the morning and at bedtime.	Helps heal gum disease.

RECOMMENDATIONS

■ Avoid spicy, oily foods as well as sugars and fermenting foods such as meat.

The best foods to eat when salivary gland disorders are present include grains, fresh fruits (except citrus), and vegetables.

■ Drink plenty of water to prevent dehydration of the gum tissues.

■ Avoid toothpastes and mouthwashes with harsh chemicals. Biotene toothpaste and mouthwash are specially formulated for dry mouth. Grace toothpaste with aloe vera and vitamin C is also recommended.

■ *See also* Salivary Glands in Part One; and Dry Mouth in Part Two.

Sensitive Teeth

See Abrasion.

Speech Problems

Speech problems can be caused by a cleft palate (see Cleft Palate and Lip in Part Two), from weakness of the muscles of the lips, tongue, and mouth, or from a variety of neurological and physical problems. Tongue thrust, the forward pressure of the tongue against the teeth, can cause lisping. Speech pathologists have found that the problem can be corrected if children get treatment before the age of seven. Ill-fitting dentures or partials can also cause a variety of speech problems, such as clicking or whistling sounds. Of course, if all the teeth are missing, speech will likely be difficult. Fractured bones in the jaw area or jawbones that have been improperly set can also present speech probems.

CONVENTIONAL TREATMENT

A dentist can put a wire behind the incisors to help break the tongue-thrusting habit. Surgery may be required to correct speech problems stemming from malformation of the membranous structures of the mouth. These structures, referred to as frenum, include the fleshy band that extends from the middle of the inside upper lip to the top of the upper two middle teeth, and the band of flesh beneath the tongue.

RECOMMENDATIONS

■ Contact a speech pathologist for help in overcoming speech problems caused by a physical weakness. (See margin note.)

■ If your speech problem is the result of an orthodontic appliance, be patient. It takes time to get used to any new applicance. Train the tongue to move correctly by reading or speaking out loud in front of a mirror.

✍ **TAKE NOTE**

If you wish to find a speech pathologist for your child, consult your *Yellow Pages* under "Speech and Language Pathologists." You can also call the American Speech-Language Hearing Association at 800–638–8255. Be aware that many states require that speech pathologists be licensed. If you have questions regarding the status of a pathologist, call your state's education department.

Stained Teeth

See Teeth, Stained.

Tartar

See Gum Disease; Plaque.

Teeth, Stained

✍ **TAKE NOTE**

Advertisements for many toothpastes claim that the products will whiten your teeth. But if you read the fine print, you'll find that the manufacturers do not actually state that the toothpaste whitens teeth, but only that it "helps" whiten or "helps whiten by removing stains."

Staining occurs on the enamel or outer surface of the teeth. Food, tobacco, and certain drugs may cause staining. Metal workers who are constantly exposed to dust containing iron, copper, or chromium commonly have stained tooth enamel. As a result of the natural process of aging, teeth may become yellowed. Ingestion of excessive amounts of fluoride—more than 2 ppm (2 parts fluoride per million parts water)—during the period when teeth are developing causes "mottled teeth."

In mild cases of mottled enamel, 50 percent of the tooth surface shows white opaque, in contrast to normal enamel, which is hard, glossy, and translucent. In moderate cases, the enamel surface has a brownish stain, and in severe cases, bands of pitting with brown or chalky stains appear on the surface of the teeth that may even crumble.

Stained teeth may be the result of long-term treatment with drugs such as tetracycline during the developmental stage of teeth. Tetracycline may cause stains ranging from yellow to brown or gray to black. It is believed that the drug binds with the calcium in the enamel. The larger the dose and the longer the drug is taken, the more severe the stains. Tetracycline should not be given to infants, children, or pregnant women unless there is a life-threatening situation.

Composite resin fillings also stain over time, and amalgam fillings stain as the result of tin oxidation. Cavities also stain teeth—the beginning stage of a cavity appears white opaque, while deeper cavities turn brown or black.

Trauma to the teeth may cause the blood vessels in the teeth, which are contained in the pulp chamber and extend through the roots via canals (see Parts of a Tooth in Part One), to rupture. The ruptured blood vessels (hematoma) are seen through the translucent enamel, giving the tooth a brown, gray, or black color.

Coffee and tea are common culprits in staining the enamel, grooves, and pits of the teeth. These dark brown stains are very difficult to remove. Tobacco, whether smoked or chewed, will produce a yellowish-brown to black discoloration. Marijuana stains manifest as dark brown to black, usually appearing as dark rings around the teeth near the gum area.

Poor oral hygiene will cause the teeth to have orange or green stains, which are actually by-products of bacteria. These types of stains are most commonly seen on children's teeth.

CONVENTIONAL TREATMENT

Thorough cleanings by a dentist or hygienist will remove most stains caused by food and tobacco, unless the stains have been present for years. Certain stains, such as those that are a result of aging, will not come off unless bleached with solutions such as hydrogen peroxide or hydrochloric acid. Enamel also has to be bleached to remove stains caused by long-term tobacco use. Bleaching the teeth may or may not remove stains caused by the drug tetracyline. Bonding and porcelain veneers are options for hard-to-remove stains. However, some forms of bonding will themselves stain after two years or longer, and bleach will have to be reapplied periodically. (For more information on bleaching and bonding teeth, see Cosmetic Dentistry in Part Three.) Stains caused by ruptured blood vessels are on the inside rather than the outside of teeth; therefore, to eliminate the stains, the teeth must be crowned or capped.

RECOMMENDATIONS

■ Practice proper oral hygiene to prevent tooth stains caused by food and tobacco.

■ Do not attempt to remove tooth stains with your fingernail or other objects.

■ Consider cosmetic options as well as preventive measures for stained or discolored teeth.

■ *See also* Cosmetic Dentistry in Part Three.

Teething

Teething, the eruption of primary teeth, usually begins when an infant is between the age of four to eight months. The bottom front teeth tend to appear first, followed by the upper middle teeth (see page 8 for the eruption sequence). Once the first tooth has erupted, a new tooth will appear approximately once a month. A child usually has a complete set of twenty baby teeth by the age of thirty months. During teething, the gums may become swollen and tender, and the baby may become irritable and restless. Discomfort due to teething may include pain.

Sometimes a bluish, watery sac called an eruption cyst appears around a tooth that is about to break through the gum surface. This requires no treatment. Eventually, the tooth will push through the gum, rupturing the cyst.

CONVENTIONAL TREATMENT

Your dentist or physician may recommend topical ointments containing lidocaine or benzocaine (e.g. Anbesol, Orajel) to numb the area. If the pain becomes severe,

✍ TAKE NOTE

Because of the stress of teething, a teething infant is more susceptible to illness. If the child has a fever higher than 100°F or a fever and diarrhea, contact your health-care provider.

the doctor may suggest giving the child an age-appropriate aspirin-free pain reliever.

HOMEOPATHIC TREATMENT

Because of their alcohol base, liquid homeopathics should not be given to children. Tablets, which have a sweet milk sugar base and can be dissolved in the mouth, are excellent for children. For infants, dissolve the tablet in water and give to the child with an eyedropper. (See Part One, Homeopathy, for additional information.)

Preparation	Directions for Use	Comments
Chamomilla 30X	Give 1 tablet hourly as needed.	Recommended to calm a restless child; use to quiet crying due to teething.
Mercurius solubilis 30X	Give 1 tablet 2 times daily as needed.	Give to infant who has sore gums and excessive salivation due to teething.

HERBAL TREATMENT

Herb	Directions for Use	Comments
Clove	Prepare as a tea (see Part Three, Using Herbs, Tea Preparation). Cool to room temperature. Strain liquid and pour into bottle or cup. Give as needed for relief.	Has soothing properties.
Licorice root	Prepare as a tea (see Part Three, Using Herbs, Tea Preparation). Cool to room temperature. Strain liquid and pour into bottle or cup. Give as needed for relief.	Has soothing properties.

RECOMMENDATIONS

■ Gently massage the baby's gums or give the infant a pacifier.

■ To relieve the pain and itching of swollen, tender gums, give the child a teething ring that has been cooled in the refrigerator or a soft, moist, cold washcloth on which to chew. Some babies prefer warmth to cold. Try both with your baby and see which is preferred, or alternate between warm and cold. Your baby may prefer a cold slice of apple, carrot, or celery for added flavor. (Be sure to give the child large, thick chunks rather than small pieces that might be a choking hazard.)

■ Topical anesthetics that contain lidocaine or benzocaine will also help soothe painful gums.

■ A low-grade fever may be the result of stress caused by teething. If, however, diarrhea is also present or the child seems unduly distressed, consult your physician.

Temporomandibular Joint Syndrome

See TMJ.

Thrush

See Yeast Infection, Oral.

Thumb-Sucking-Related Problems

The sucking reflex is normal and healthy in babies. However, if the habit persists once the child is on solid food, attention should be given to help stop the habit. Sucking of fingers by older children usually supplies psychological comfort, but if the habit continues once the permanent teeth erupt, problems may result.

Thumb-sucking causes the teeth to develop abnormally, and produces the open bite shown in the margin figure. Sores may develop on the finger or fingers that are most frequently sucked. If the child continues this habit, as he or she gets older, the sucked fingers may eventually become deformed.

The most suitable time to help a child break this habit is between four and seven years of age. During this time, it is still possible to prevent serious damage to the permanent teeth. If thumb-sucking continues after the adult teeth begin to erupt, the teeth may become permanently displaced.

HOMEOPATHIC TREATMENT

Because of their alcohol base, liquid homeopathic preparations should not be given to children. Tablets, which have a sweet milk sugar base and can be dissolved in the mouth, are excellent for children. For infants, dissolve the tablet in water, and give it to the child in an eyedropper. (See Part One, Homeopathy, for additional information.)

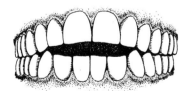

Open Bite
Result of habitual thumb-sucking.

Preparation	Directions for Use	Comments
Ambra grisia 3X	Take 1 tablet daily.	Helpful for calming nervous children.

RECOMMENDATIONS

■ When the child is younger than four years old, gently pull the finger out of his or her mouth whenever you notice that it's being sucked.

■ The most successful treatment with a child older than four is to talk to him or her in a calm, friendly manner and explain what can happen if the habit is not broken. Show the child the figure on page 139. Do not use threats, but educate the child. He or she should be ready to participate in the process without being forced. Explain that if the child is ready to break the habit, you are ready to help, and together you will be successful. For further information, contact your dentist.

■ Keep a record of days that your child has not sucked his or her thumb or fingers by marking them with stars on a calendar. At the end of a certain number of days in a row without thumb-sucking (number of days to be determined by you), the child should get a reward. If the finger or thumb is sucked, the stars must be started again from day one.

■ During the day, a bandage can be placed on the finger as a reminder not to suck it. Soaking the bandage in hot pepper or garlic oil may also help. At night, a sock or mitten can be worn on the hand or hands to deter the child from thumb-sucking.

■ If there is no change after two or three months, consult an orthodontist. He or she may provide an appliance that will discourage finger-sucking. These appliances are not very pleasant to the child and should be considered only if all else has failed.

■ *See also* Orthodontic Techniques in Part Three.

TMJ (Temporomandibular Joint Syndrome)

Problems related to the jaw are among the most misdiagnosed conditions in the body. Aches in the face, head, neck, shoulders, and back may be the result of jaw misalignments, fractures, or other jaw problems. One such problem is temporo-mandibular joint syndrome, commonly known as TMJ. An estimated 10 million Americans suffer from TMJ, which occurs when the temporomandibular joint (the hinge that connects the upper and lower jaw) becomes misaligned. This misalign-ment causes degeneration of the jaw joint, resulting in muscle and joint pain in the jaw area.

The correct relationship of the jaw to the head is seen in the figure on page 141. Also shown is a close-up of the temporomandibular joint. There are two such joints—one on the right side and one on the left side of the head. Each joint is surrounded by a saclike sheath that contains synovial fluid, which lubricates and nourishes the joint. At each end of the lower jaw, there is a knoblike structure called a *condyle*. Condyles, which are found throughout the body, are attached to muscles that join bones to nearby bones. Mounted on top of each condyle is a *disc*—a cushion made of cartilage that sits between the joint and its socket. In the jaw, this disc

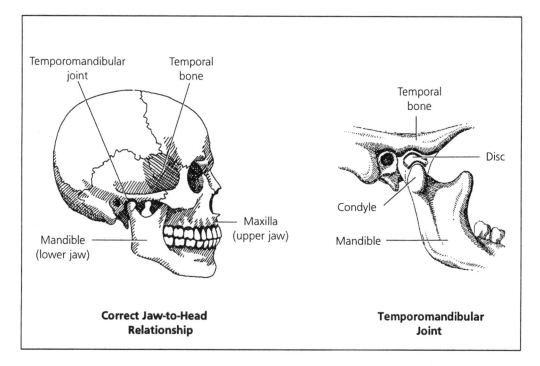

Correct Jaw-to-Head Relationship

Temporomandibular Joint

moves with the condyle and prevents it from hitting the temporal bone. When the disc is worn away or abnormally placed, the jaw becomes misaligned.

The margin figure shows a temporomandibular joint in which the disc has degenerated. Notice how the condyle is making contact with the temporal bone above it; there is no space in the socket. In addition to this condition causing jaw pain, pain from TMJ commonly radiates to other areas of the head and neck. And since this joint is located in front of the ear, TMJ may also cause pain or discomfort in the ears, eyes, and sinuses.

Under normal conditions, the jaw joint is capable of performing three motions with ease. It can open and close, move backward and forward, and shift from side to side. Several factors can interfere with proper jaw movements and lead to TMJ. These factors include trauma to the head, tooth clenching or grinding, poor posture, missing teeth, or poorly placed fillings, crowns, bridges, or dentures.

Problems that are characteristic of TMJ include:

- *Headaches.* Depending on the severity of the disorder, headaches may be mild and intermittent or severe and constant (as in a migraine headache). The pain usually affects one or both sides of the temples, and the top or base of the skull. You may feel as if there is a painful band around your head. Areas where pain radiates are indicated in the figure on page 142.

- *Eye aches.* Pain and pressure deep behind the eyes is a common complaint.

- *Ear disturbances.* Ringing in the ears (tinnitus), swishing noises, and/or a "stuffed" sensation are common symptoms related to the ear. Pain when infection is not present is also a symptom.

- *Clicking, popping, or grating noises.* When the jaw opens or closes, these noises may be heard in varying degrees from one or both sides of the jaw.

- *Neck, shoulder, and backaches.* Pain and stiffness in the neck, shoulders, and back are sometimes accompanied by numbness and tingling that runs down the arms and through the hands.

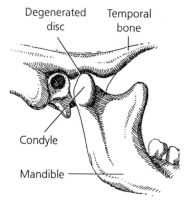

Temporomandibular Joint with TMJ
*Note the lack of socket space due to degenerated disc.

141

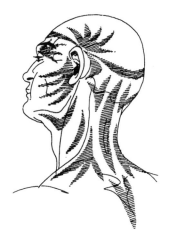

**Areas of Pain
Caused by TMJ**

■ *Lockjaw.* Opening and closing the jaw may be difficult due to pain or interference from something locking the jaw in one position. Sometimes the jaw needs to deviate to one side in order to open, rather than opening straight up and straight down.

■ *Sinus pain and toothaches.* Pressure in the sinus area and toothaches that cannot be traced to any cavities or other problems may be related to TMJ disorders.

■ *Dizziness.* Due to the relative position of the jaw joint and the ear, pressure in this area may cause dizziness or loss of equilibrium.

A jaw imbalance that has existed since birth may be aggravated by orthodontia if the teeth are straightened but the bite is not adjusted properly. Poor dental habits also tend to cause jaw problems. Chewing on one side of the mouth rather than on both sides, sucking the thumb, swallowing improperly by pushing the tongue against the teeth, internalizing stress by clenching or grinding the teeth (bruxism), and constantly chewing gum may all cause TMJ disorders.

TMJ disorders may manifest in three areas of the jaw—the muscles, joints, and discs. If the disorder affects the muscles that directly control the jaw joints, pain may result from chewing. However, the pain may radiate in the head, neck, and shoulders, as shown in margin figure. This form of the disorder is called myofascial pain dysfunction (MPD). Muscle spasms are frequently present with myofascial pain. MPD may affect one or more muscle groups. The most common cause of MPD is tension and stress. Tension triggers muscle spasms, causing pain, creating more anxiety and tension, causing more spasms and pain, and the cycle continues.

Inflammation of the jaw joints is another type of TMJ disorder. There are two forms of inflammation of the jaw joint. Capsulitis or synovitis involves the inflammation of the capsule lining. Retrodiscitis is an inflammation of the area located behind the disc. Inflammation of the jaw joints can be caused by trauma, infection, constant spasms of the chewing muscles, and arthritis, which is discussed below. For a variety of reasons, there may be displacement of the disc, causing the third form of TMJ disorder.

Before treatment for TMJ is considered, the cause of the jaw imbalance must be determined. The main causes are:

■ *Stress and anxiety.* Sometimes, when feelings are internalized, grinding and clenching the teeth become a habit. Teeth become worn down and the muscles involved in chewing become fatigued, causing pain. Eventually the disc may become displaced, leading to arthritis of the jaw joints. If a person who grinds his or her teeth is unaware of the damage this causes and does not break the habit, treatment will be virtually useless. These individuals will seek ongoing treatment with little relief, not realizing they are contributing to the problem.

■ *Bad habits.* Poor posture, carrying heavy things on one's shoulder for long periods of time, wearing high-heeled shoes, talking on the telephone while holding the receiver between the shoulder and the ear, and placing pressure under the chin or face with a fist or the hands will all burden the muscles involved with the jaw joint. Mouth-breathing and tongue-thrusting are other habits that may also damage the jaw joints.

■ *Trauma.* Injuries to the head and neck, such as those from a direct blow or whiplash, may cause dislocation, fractures, strains, and tears of the jaw muscles. Severe trauma may also cause internal bleeding in the disc area. Subsequently, hard, fibrous tissue forms in the joint, causing permanent hardening or stiffening (ankylosis). Opening the mouth too wide when yawning, or keeping the mouth open for long dental surgeries may also traumatize the jaw.

■ *Malocclusion*. Bad bite may cause the total mechanism of the jaw to go into an unbalanced position. Some of the teeth and the muscles used for chewing may have to work harder to compensate for others that may be fatigued and weakened due to the imbalance. This situation can be compared to someone who may have to limp on one foot for a long period of time. Eventually, the muscles from one side will have to carry the load for both sides, causing fatigue and pain to the overworked muscle group.

■ *Arthritis*. A disease characterized by inflammation and pain in body joints, arthritis may involve one or both joints of the jaw. Arthritis affects almost 90 percent of the United States population between the ages of twenty and sixty.

Rheumatoid arthritis is a chronic systemic disease of unknown cause. Individuals with this disease complain of pain, heat, and swelling around the joints. Stiffness of the neck and jaw have also been reported, limiting movement and making it impossible to close the mouth. Initially, there may be no pain; however, chewing, talking, and clenching the teeth will exacerbate the inflammation, eventually causing pain. In cases of advanced and severe rheumatoid arthritis, deformity of the face may result as parts of the jaw joint, especially the condyle, may be resorbed or dissolved. This will cause the bite to change so that only the back teeth touch.

Gouty arthritis occurs when there is an excessive level of uric acid crystals in the blood. The abnormal level results from a defect in body chemistry and is accompanied by inflammation and pain. When gout, which occurs more often in men, affects the jaws, the individual complains of pain on movement and a sandpaper-like grinding sound from the area of the jaw joint. As uric acid increases in concentration, the symptoms usually become worse.

Osteoarthritis, rarely seen in children and young adults, is caused by wear of the body's joints. Individuals who lead a sedentary and inactive life, void of physical exercise, are more prone to osteoarthritis, which is seen most often in the elderly. There are two types of osteoarthritis—primary and secondary. Primary osteoarthritis is a degenerative disease of a healthy joint. The condition occurs gradually, and stiffness and pain are common complaints. The secondary type results from an injury, infection, or an old fracture. Tooth grinding and clenching are common causes of osteoarthritis in the jaw joint. By placing overloaded stress and pressure on the joint, the condyle and other bones of the joints eventually change shape and dry out the lubricating fluids. Bone begins to grind against bone, causing severe pain. X-rays may show the joint as flattened and irregular with bony spurs and sharp edges. Sometimes, these bony spurs break off and move about inside the joint space. The disc itself may tear, become thin, and detach from the fibers holding it in its proper place. Arthritic conditions can be aggravated by malocclusion, which in itself does not cause any form of arthritis.

You can tell if you are grinding or clenching your teeth by focusing on your jaws and noting if they feel sore, particularly upon waking. Grinding and clenching the teeth causes constant muscle contraction, interfering with circulation; lactic acid builds up, and sore muscles result. Your teeth should touch only when you are chewing or swallowing. When your jaw is at rest, the teeth should be apart.

To determine if your jaw joint has been pushed out of its normal position, place your pinky or little finger in your ears and gently press forward. Very slowly open and close your mouth. If you hear clicking, popping, or grinding noises in your ear(s), the joints are not in the correct position. Depending on the degree of imbalance, the noises may be slight or very loud, and may be noticed in one ear or both. The noise may be heard upon opening or closing the mouth or when chewing. With normal movements, the jaw and the disc move together. Noise occurs when the disc is pushed out of its proper position over the condyle. When the jaw snaps back into position underneath the disc, movement continues without noise. If you hear any sounds, it is advisable to have your jaw joints evaluated by a dentist who is trained to diagnose and treat TMJ disorders.

If clicking is heard when the jaw is just beginning to open, the condition is usually easier to treat than when the click occurs with widest openings. In the former case, the ligaments holding the disc in place have not been stretched too severely, and may be able to regain their original position (recapturing the disc) with proper treatment.

In addition to TMJ, there are other causes of jaw problems. Osteomyelitis of the jaw, an infection of bone and bone marrow, produces severe pain and high fever. This is commonly caused by the spread of infection when a tooth is pulled. Jaw pain and soreness may also result from prolonged dental treatment, when the mouth is kept open for hours. This pain may remain for weeks. Another cause of jawbone destruction is radiation therapy for cancer of the face, head, and neck. Destroyed bone may be restored with plastic and maxillofacial surgery.

CONVENTIONAL TREATMENT

The treatment of TMJ disorders involves a multidisciplinary approach. Besides a dentist, a chiropractor, nutritionist, physical therapist, biofeedback therapist, osteopath, and ear, nose, and throat physician may need to be consulted.

It is important to note that there may be no total cure for TMJ disorders. Symptoms can be eliminated successfully; however, you must realize this is a weak area. If TMJ is aggravated by trauma, yawning too wide, poor posture, eating hard foods on one side, clenching or grinding the teeth, etc., the symptoms will return.

Your dentist may recommend a bite plate or repositioning splint, which is effective for separating the jaws. The bite plate (or night guard, if it is worn only at night) is usually made for those who clench or grind their teeth; it allows you to close your mouth where you feel most comfortable. Made of either a hard or soft acrylic, a bite plate is worn on either the top or bottom teeth. The repositioning splint is a hard acrylic plate worn on either the top or bottom teeth, or on the back teeth only. This splint has contours of the opposing teeth, so that when you close your mouth, shallow contours on the splint guide the teeth to the correct contact point, thereby repositioning the jaw. Depending on the degree of imbalance, you may be told to wear the splint for specific periods during the day or night, or to leave it in constantly. If you wear the appliance constantly, it is usually for a period of up to six months, with weekly adjustments by the dentist.

As the symptoms taper off, you will decrease the amount of time you wear the splint. After the symptoms have been eliminated, the dentist will recommend several options. One is to wear a permanent repositioning splint, mostly during the day for an indefinite period of time. Or the dentist may recommend you wear the splint only when the joints become aggravated. Another option is to correct malocclusion by adjusting the bite with new fillings, crowns, or orthodontics, or by selectively smoothing surfaces of teeth.

To treat muscle pain, your dentist may use ultrasound or electrogalvanic stimulation (EGS) for heat application. Ultrasound generates high frequency sound waves that heat tissue and penetrate deep under the skin. EGS passes mild electric currents that produce heat therapy to muscle fibers, increasing blood flow.

Dentists or physical therapists may spray the affected muscles with an anesthetic such as fluorimethane, which helps relieve muscle spasm and pain. Repeated use of the sprays along with other suggested methods of treatment will sustain improvement.

For severe muscle pain, a muscle relaxer such as Norflex may be prescribed, along with tranquilizers and pain medications. Corticosteroid and local anesthetic injections also may provide temporary relief from pain and tenderness. Surgery may be recommended, but only as a last resort (unless there is a definite structural abnormality due to a dislocated disc, osteoarthritis, or a discrepancy in size and shape of the upper and lower jaws).

Osteopathic physicians may be consulted to adjust cranial and facial bones. Physical therapists can massage muscle tissues and recommend specific exercises for weakened muscles.

NUTRITIONAL SUPPLEMENTS

Supplement	Directions for Use	Comments
Calcium	Take 1500 mg daily.	Helps improve muscle function.
Coenzyme Q-10	Take 60 mg daily.	Helps improve circulation.
Folic acid	Take 400 mcg daily.	Useful for treatment of anxiety and depression.
Magnesium	Take 750 mg daily.	Works with calcium to improve muscle function.
Vitamin B complex	Take 100 mg daily.	Important for stress management.
Vitamin C	Take 2000 mg daily.	Helps repair connective tissue involved with jaw joint attachment.

HOMEOPATHIC TREATMENT

Dissolve the tablets under your tongue. Do not eat or drink for fifteen minutes prior to or after taking medication. (See Part One, Homeopathy, for additional information.)

Preparation	Directions for Use	Comments
Aconite 30X	Take 1 tablet 3 times daily.	Use for relief from anxiety, nervousness, and restlessness; relieves stiff, painful neck.
Ammonium carbonica 6X	Take 1 tablet 3 times daily.	Helps jaw pain when chewing.
Arnica 30X	Take 1 tablet 3 times daily.	Indicated for sore muscles and sprains.
Hepar sulphuris 30X	Take 1 tablet 3 times daily.	Decreases anxiety; lessens pain upon opening and closing the jaw.

Rhamnus califomica 6X	Take 1 tablet every 4 hours.	Aids in relief of muscle pain and swollen joints.
Xerophyllum 6X	Take 1 tablet hourly.	Helps decrease headache and pressure in sinuses.

HERBAL TREATMENT

Herb	Directions for Use	Comments
Arnica and black cohosh	Prepare together as tea (see Part Three, Using Herbs, Tea Preparation) or take 250-mg tablet of each once a day as needed.	Helps relieve cramps, pain, muscle tension, and muscle sprains.
Comfrey, burdock, and marigold	Prepare together as tea (see Part Three, Using Herbs, Tea Preparation). Soak a washcloth in the warm tea and apply to sore and painful muscles as needed.	Helps relieve muscle pain.
Lobelia	Prepare as tea (see Part Three, Using Herbs, Tea Preparation). Drink as needed.	A good relaxant.
Lobelia, black cohosh, skullcap, cayenne, marigold, and myrrh	Prepare together as tea (see Part Three, Using Herbs, Tea Preparation). Drink as needed.	Helps relieve jaw pain.

RECOMMENDATIONS

■ For painful, sore muscles, alternating moist heat and cold applications are helpful. Cold helps relax muscle spasms and numbs pain. Heat, on the other hand, increases the flow of oxygen to the tissues by dilating blood vessels and increasing blood flow. Some people, however, find that they respond better to heat; others, to cold. Try both, and see which feels better.

■ Massage your face, neck, and shoulders to help relax sore muscles and improve circulation.

■ When pain is present in the jaw area and while you are being treated, stick with a soft, bland diet. Foods high in fiber, steamed vegetables, juices, and water are best. Stay away from hard foods that cause your jaws to work a lot. Avoid caffeine, which is found in coffee, tea, colas, and chocolate. Caffeine increases muscle tension and makes the nervous system more sensitive, signaling more pain.

■ Treat your sore jaw as you would a sore ankle. If your ankle were sprained, you would try to stay off it. While your jaw is sore, try not to open your mouth too wide. Open only as far as is comfortable. Keep your jaw in a relaxed position—a position in which your teeth do not touch. Place your tongue on the roof of your mouth, and keep your lips closed. Breathe through your nose. The only time your teeth should touch is when you are chewing or swallowing.

■ Before retiring at night, take a hot shower or bath and gently stretch your neck and back muscles to relax them.

■ Exercises for the jaw are very helpful. While looking in the mirror, place your tongue on the roof of your mouth; slowly practice opening and closing your mouth. Keeping your tongue on the roof of your mouth allows you to open and close your mouth without swinging your jaw.

■ Practice proper posture at all times, whether sitting or walking.

■ *See also* The Jaw in Part One; and Acupressure in Part Three.

Tongue-Related Problems

Tongue-related problems may be divided into three categories: tongue inflammation or "glossitis," disorders arising in the tongue itself, and disorders resulting from other conditions existing in the body.

The cause of glossitis is not known. When glossitis is present, the normal hairlike projections on the upper surface of the tongue (papillae) disappear. The surface of the tongue takes on a bald appearance and may have a purplish red color. The whole tongue may become painful and sore. A burning sensation may be experienced, and swallowing may become difficult. In the condition called geographic tongue, patches of the tongue lose the papillae, leaving uneven borders of white or yellow. The patches may heal, and other areas of the tongue may lose the papillae and appear bald. This condition is also referred to as migratory glossitis since there is the illusion that the patches are moving. Most of the time, people don't even know that they have the condition unless they eat spicy or acidic foods, which leave a burning sensation on the bald areas.

Usually, individuals with geographic tongue also have fissured tongue. This is a congenital condition in which a deep trenchlike area runs along the top surface of the tongue. The depth of the fissure can vary along its length. Food may collect in the deep fissures, causing inflammation. Spicy or acidic foods will cause a burning sensation. There is no treatment for fissured tongue except to keep the area clean by brushing it and using a mouthwash.

Hairy tongue is usually seen in individuals who irritate the tongue with tobacco use. The condition is harmless, except that bacteria may harbor on the "hairy" surface, causing infection. The hairlike areas are due to the papillae's becoming longer and darker. There is no treatment for hairy tongue.

Enlargement of the tongue is associated with a number of congenital diseases. These include lymphangioma, a benign tumor of the lymph vessels that is seen early in life and can be surgically treated. Down's syndrome is another congenital condition in which the tongue is enlarged. The tongue may become so large that it is difficult to close the mouth. Neurofibromatosis (von Rochlinghausen's disease) is another disorder in which tumors form in nerve tissue. Neurofibromas may also occur on the tongue, giving it an enlarged appearance. Although the tumors can be surgically removed, they commonly reappear.

Certain infections such as hepatitis may produce a bitter taste in the mouth, while other disorders such as candidiasis may cause a total loss of taste. Many salivary gland disorders cause dry mouth and an inability to taste foods. And many drugs alter the taste buds.

Nutritional deficiencies may also cause disorders of the tongue. This is especially common in the elderly. Older individuals who have been chronically ill and malnourished often have strawberry tongue (a tongue that is deep red in color). Folic acid anemia—caused by alcoholism, poor diet, or the use of certain medications—as well as pernicious anemia—a serious blood disease caused by vitamin B_{12} deficiency—are commonly associated with glossitis.

CONVENTIONAL TREATMENT

Your physician will treat nutritional deficiencies according to the particular deficiency. Infections will be treated with the appropriate antibiotic.

NUTRITIONAL SUPPLEMENT

Supplement	Directions for Use	Comments
Folic acid	Take 400 mcg daily or as prescribed by your physician.	Helps prevent or reverse the glossitis associated with folic acid anemia.
Garlic	Take two 250-mg tablets 3 times daily.	Has natural antibiotic properties.
Iron	Take 18 mg daily.	Prevents iron-deficiency anemia.
Vitamin B complex	Take 100 mg daily.	Helps prevent glossitis.

HOMEOPATHIC TREATMENT

Preparation	Directions for Use	Comments
Arsenicum album 6X	Take 1 tablet daily.	Helps relieve dry tongue and burning sensation.
Ignatia 6X	Take 1 tablet 2 times daily.	Improves function of taste buds.

HERBAL TREATMENT

Herb	Directions for Use	Comments
Alfalfa, red clover, and burdock	Prepare a tea (see Part Three, Using Herbs, Tea Preparation) using all or a combination of these herbs. Drink 2–3 cups a day or take tablets as directed on package.	Important in rebuilding the blood.

RECOMMENDATIONS

■ Brushing the tongue when hairy tongue or geographic tongue is present will help prevent infections.

■ Tobacco use should be discontinued with hairy tongue.

■ Eating raisins, prunes, dried apricots, wheat germ, and brewer's yeast will help strengthen blood.

■ *See also* The Tongue in Part One; and Dry Mouth; Yeast Infection in Part Two.

Tongue-Thrusting

See Speech Problems.

Tooth, Loss of

Teeth can be lost due to gum disease, cavities, failed fillings or root canals, radiation therapy, systemic diseases, or injury. Teeth may also be intentionally removed for orthodontic reasons, as when teeth are too crowded.

When all the teeth are present, the forces of chewing are distributed evenly. Once teeth are lost, the equilibrium of the mouth is compromised. Chewing becomes impeded as the remaining teeth have to bear the forces of chewing for the missing teeth. Due to the excessive force on the remaining teeth, the bone may become weak and the teeth may become loose. Speaking may become difficult if teeth are missing or if the bone becomes weak.

When a tooth is lost, the adjacent tooth and the opposing tooth will eventually begin to shift, since every tooth is dependent on every other tooth to maintain its normal position and function. Many times, pulling a tooth causes new problems that may affect the teeth, gums, and bone.

When teeth are lost on one side of the mouth, the tendency is to chew on the side with more teeth. This, however, is not a good thing. The muscles on the used side of the mouth will be overworked, causing overcontraction; muscle degeneration will occur on the unused side. Temporomandibular joint disorders are likely to result. (See TMJ in Part Two.)

It is very important to replace lost teeth as soon as possible. Until you get replacement teeth, be sure to chew on both sides of your mouth. However, try to limit yourself to soft foods. Chewing hard foods will cause the bony ridge where the teeth used to be to become flat, making it very difficult to place dentures or bridges.

FIRST AID

✚ Knocked-out teeth may be successfully replaced in the tooth's socket, if done within 30 minutes of the tooth's falling out. Never hold the tooth by the root. Rinse any dirt or blood off the tooth with cold water, replace it in the tooth socket, and get to the dentist immediately. If you cannot see the dentist in less than 30 minutes, keep the tooth wrapped in a moist cloth or gauze, place it in a container of milk, or leave it under your tongue until you are treated.

CONVENTIONAL TREATMENT

When teeth are lost, replacements should be considered as soon as possible since no one can predict how soon problems may occur with the remaining teeth. Options for tooth replacement include bridges, dentures, and implants. (See Implants; Prosthodontic Techniques in Part Three.)

NUTRITIONAL SUPPLEMENTS

Supplement	Directions for Use	Comments
Beta-cartone	Take 10,000 IU daily.	Helps heal gum tissue.
Calcium	Take 1500 mg daily.	Important for healthy bone.

| Magnesium | Take 750 mg daily. | Works with calcium to strengthen bone. |
| Vitamin C | Take 1500 mg daily. | Helps maintain healthy gums. |

HOMEOPATHIC TREATMENT

Dissolve the tablets under your tongue. Do not eat or drink for fifteen minutes prior to or after taking medication. (See Part One, Homeopathy, for additional information.)

Preparation	Directions for Use	Comments
Ammonium carbonica 6X	Take 1 tablet 3 times daily.	Indicated for pain upon chewing.
Arnica 30X	Take 1 tablet hourly.	Helps relieve pain in jaw joint caused by chewing on one side of the mouth.
Lachesis 30X	Take 1 tablet daily.	Helpful for swollen, spongy gums.

HERBAL TREATMENT

Herb	Directions for Use	Comments
Aloe vera	Place gel on a cotton-tipped swab (see Part Three, Using Herbs, Application Preparation) and rub on the gums. Do not eat or drink for at least 1 hour after applying the gel.	Helpful for sore gums.
Arnica	Apply cream (available at health-food stores) topically to sore area.	Helpful for a jaw that is sore due to chewing on one side of the mouth.
Chamomile	Prepare as a tea (see Part Three, Using Herbs, Tea Preparation). Drink 2 to 3 cups daily.	Promotes relaxation.
Chamomile and goldenseal	Prepare together as a mouthwash (see Part Three, Using Herbs, Mouthwash Preparation). Use as needed.	Soothes painful gums.

RECOMMENDATIONS

■ Until missing teeth are replaced, avoid the tendency to chew only on the side of the mouth with the most teeth. Chew soft foods, using both sides of the mouth.

■ It is important to understand the advantages of saving teeth and the disadvantages of losing teeth. In the long run, it is better—more cost effective and simpler—to save teeth, even though it may appear simpler to pull them.

■ *See also* Trauma to Children's Teeth in Part Two.

Tooth Decay

See Cavities.

Tooth-Extraction-Related Problems

See Dry Socket; Impacted Teeth in Part One; and Surgery; Tooth Extraction in Part Three.

Tooth Grinding

See Bruxism.

Tooth Sensitivity

See Abrasion.

Toothache

At some time in their lives, most people will experience a toothache. A toothache may be the result of a cavity, a gum infection, a crack in the tooth, pressure from orthodontic treatment, or a normal reaction to dental treatment.

Occasionally, a toothache is the result of something as simple as trapped food between teeth. In this case, the problem is actually with the irritated gums and the supporting tissue, not the tooth. Usually the pain is minimal and the tooth is sore to biting forces. The good news is that this situation can be corrected rather easily and without a trip to the dentist's office. Simply rinse your mouth with warm water to loosen and remove any foreign matter. Then use dental floss or a water-irrigating

7 Things You Can Do to Relieve Toothache Pain

Tooth pain is a sign that something is wrong. A toothache may develop due to a number of reasons—a cavity, a gum infection, a crack in the tooth, pressure from orthodontic treatment, or a normal reaction to recent dental treatment. Pain from a toothache can radiate from a specific tooth, or it can be more generalized, affecting a wider area of the mouth.

With any tooth pain, the first thing you should do is seek professional treatment. In the meantime, there are several things you can do yourself to minimize the pain:

1. For temporary relief, treat the tooth topically with an over-the-counter ointment containing lidocaine or benzocaine, such as Campho-Phenique, Orajel, or Anbesol. Or soak a cotton ball with clove or wintergreen oil and place it directly on the sore tooth.

2. Avoid hard, chewy foods, as well as very hot or cold foods or drinks.

3. Depending on your individual preference, take an over-the-counter pain reliever, including one that contains acetaminophen, aspirin, or ibuprofen. Advil and Motrin are two of these products that may also reduce inflammation. *Aspirin and other analgesics should never be applied topically to the area surrounding a sore tooth; these products contain strong acids that may burn the gum tissues.*

4. Drink warm chamomile tea, which helps relieve pain and headache and reduce fever, or drink warm echinacea tea, which has antibiotic and anti-inflammatory properties. (To prepare herbal teas, see Using Herbs, Tea Preparation, in Part Three.)

5. Warm salt-water rinses or a solution of warm salt water mixed with a tablespoon of aloe vera gel may reduce gum irritation and tooth pain.

6. For toothache from an impacted tooth, a small piece of ice placed over the swollen gums may bring temporary relief. *Please note: with this exception, extremes of hot or cold should not be applied directly to a sore tooth or any other area within the mouth. Mouthwashes, salves, and ointments should be lukewarm before they are applied. Even teas should be warm—not hot—before they are taken.*

7. To reduce swelling and jaw pain from tooth extraction, oral surgery, temporo-mandibular joint disorder (TMJ), or trauma, place an ice pack outside the jaw area in 5 to 15 minute intervals for 2 to 3 hours. This will help reduce swelling and relieve pain. Several hours later or even the next day, you can apply hot compresses to the area for further pain relief. *Remember, these applications are for outside the jaw area only. Extremes of hot and cold should not be used for pain control inside the mouth.*

device to remove any food that is trapped between the teeth. (See Oral Hygiene in Part Three.)

Sometimes, the pain from a toothache is intermittent. This form of pain is most deceiving, because the individual may tend to ignore it, thinking it will go away as it has before. However, any sign of pain—constant or intermittent—is the body's means of telling us that something is wrong. If pain is felt only once, perhaps nothing more than a minor trauma—chewing a hard form of food—caused the pain. However, if there is any kind of pattern to the pain, then immediate treatment should be administered.

The dentist is the only one qualified, with the help of x-rays, observation, and asking appropriate questions, of diagnosing the cause of the tooth pain. If a cavity is the cause, the decayed tooth tissue must be removed and a filling must be placed to restore the tooth. Filling materials may include amalgam or silver, composite resins, porcelain, or gold. (See Filling a Cavity in Part Three.) When the damage to a tooth covers a large area, a filling may not be enough to restore the tooth, and enamel may be replaced with a cap or crown. (See Cosmetic Dentistry in Part Three.) If the cavity has reached the nerve of the tooth, severe pain, especially to hot and cold, may be felt. In this case, root canal therapy or tooth extraction may be indicated. (See Endodontic Techniques; Tooth Extraction in Part Three.)

A crack in a tooth may be felt as pressure and pain when chewing; it is often accompanied by sensitivity to hot and cold. Initially the pain may be weak and occasional, eventually becoming more pronounced and frequent. If the crack affects the enamel and dentin of a tooth, a cap or crown is often the best choice of treatment. However, if the crack is severe, root canal therapy or tooth extraction may be necessary. (See Broken, Cracked, or Chipped Teeth in Part Two.) Also, it is important to determine the cause of the crack to prevent other teeth from cracking in the future.

Another cause of tooth pain is from new cavities that have formed under old fillings or crowns. In these cases, the old filling or crown is removed, and the cavity is cleaned. A new filling or crown is then placed to restore the tooth.

A gum infection may sometimes be felt as a toothache. If you have a history of gum disease and notice bleeding and swollen gums surrounding a tooth, seek immediate treatment. Left untreated, the gum infection will eventually affect the tooth, which may then require root canal therapy as well as gum treatments. (See Gum Disease in Part Two.) Sometimes, a sinus infection may translate into pain that is felt in the upper back teeth (molars). Until the infection is eliminated, the toothache will not go away.

CONVENTIONAL TREATMENT

Tooth pain is usually a sign that something is wrong. An early visit to the dentist for diagnosis is a wise decision that may prevent lengthy, expensive treatments. Depending on the cause or type of pain, the dentist will make the appropriate treatment suggestions.

Everyone tolerates pain differently. In some individuals, pain produces anxiety, which, in turn, seems to increase the pain. Over-the-counter pain relievers are available, including those that contain acetaminophen, aspirin, and ibuprofen. Advil and Motrin are two of these products that may also reduce inflammation.

NUTRITIONAL SUPPLEMENTS

Supplement	Directions for Use	Comments
Calcium	Take 1200 mg daily.	Important in regulation of nerve impulses.
Magnesium	Take 600 mg daily.	Assists in calcium uptake.
Vitamin C	Take 1000 mg daily.	Prolongs effects of aspirin.

Vitamin E	Take 400 IU daily.	Powerful antioxidant; improves circulation; helps repair damaged tissues.

HOMEOPATHIC TREATMENT

Dissolve the tablets under your tongue. Do not eat or drink for fifteen minutes prior to or after taking medication. (See Part One, Homeopathy, for additional information.)

Preparation	Directions for Use	Comments
Calcarea carbonica 6X	Take 1 tablet every 15 minutes, decreasing to 1 tablet every 2 hours depending on pain.	Helps relieve tooth pain from hot and cold.
Hypericum 30X	Take 1 tablet hourly as needed, for one day.	Helps relieve severe tooth pain following root canal therapy or oral surgery.
Mercurius hydrargyrum 6X	Take 1 tablet hourly as needed.	Helps relieve pain from gum or bone infection that is worse at night or when lying down.
Rhus toxicodendron 30X	Take 1 tablet hourly as needed.	Helps relieve sore gums and pain from loose teeth.

HERBAL TREATMENT

Herbs	Directions for Use	Comments
Black cohosh	Prepare as a tea (see Part Three, Using Herbs, Tea Preparation). Drink at room temperature as needed, or take capsules or tablets as directed on package.	Helps relieve pain. *Do not take if pregnant.*
Catnip	Prepare as a tea (see Part Three, Using Herbs, Tea Preparation). Drink as needed, or take capsules or tablets as directed on package.	Helps lower anxiety.
Chamomile	Prepare as a tea (see Part Three, Using Herbs, Tea Preparation). Drink as needed, or take capsules or tablets as directed on package.	Helps relieve pain and headache, and reduce fever.
Clove oil	Place on cotton-tipped swab and rub on the affected tooth.	Helps relieve pain.
Comfrey root	Prepare as a tea (see Part Three, Using Herbs, Tea Preparation.) Drink as needed, or take capsules or tablets as directed on package.	Helps relieve pain and cramps. *May cause liver damage if taken regularly for longer than three months.*
Echinacea	Prepare as a tea (see Part Three, Using Herbs, Tea Preparation). Drink as needed, or take capsules or tablets as directed on package.	Has antibiotic and anti-inflammatory properties.
Goldenseal	Prepare as a tea or mouthwash (see Part Three, Using Herbs). Drink the tea or use as a mouthwash as needed.	Has antibiotic and anti-inflammatory properties. *Use only as needed. Long-term use may disrupt bacterial content in the colon.*

Wintergreen oil	Place on cotton-tipped swab and rub on the affected tooth.	Helps relieve pain.

RECOMMENDATIONS

■ Seek treatment for tooth pain as soon as possible.

■ Avoid hard, chewy foods, as well as very hot or cold foods or drinks.

■ For sore gums, rinse your mouth with a solution of warm salt water and a tablespoon of aloe vera gel.

■ *See also* Broken, Cracked, or Chipped Teeth; Cavities; Pain and Anxiety; TMJ in Part Two; and First Aid in Part Three.

Tori

See Cysts and Tumors.

Trauma to Adults' Teeth

See Broken, Cracked, or Chipped Teeth; Tooth, Loss of.

Trauma to Children's Teeth

Due to the activities in which children engage, trauma to the mouth is not unusual. In fact, among the most common problems associated with children's teeth are those caused by accidents. Fractures to either the crown or root surfaces can occur when a child bumps into objects, falls down, or is injured during sports. The child should be taken to the dentist as soon as possible to determine the extent of the damage.

A crack or fracture may or may not cause damage to the nerve of the tooth. The dentist will determine if the nerve has been affected. If it has, the nerve should be treated unless the involved tooth is a baby tooth that will come out soon. Nerve treatment may require root canal therapy. For baby teeth, a modified form of root canal called a pulpotomy is performed. (See Endodontic Techniques in Part Three.) Sometimes nerve damage does not show up immediately. The dentist will probably check the nerve every three months.

FIRST AID

✚ If your child is in pain, give him or her an aspirin-free, age-appropriate pain reliever.

✚ Tell your child to avoid chewing with the cracked tooth. Do not give your child foods or liquids that are very hot or cold.

✚ Clean the wound, unless a splinter or other object is imbedded in the area. If this is the case, wait and see a professional.

✚ Apply pressure with gauze to stop any bleeding.

✚ If possible, keep any part of the tooth that is broken, especially if it is a gold or porcelain filling, which can sometimes be recemented to the tooth.

155

If a trauma causes a baby tooth to be pushed out of position, wait until the pain has stopped and place gentle pressure on the tooth to move it back to its proper place. Stop immediately if this action causes pain. Teach the child to periodically place pressure on the tooth with the tongue or lip, depending on the direction the tooth was displaced.

Some trauma will cause a baby tooth to recede into the gums. Do not be alarmed. Keep the area clean with a cotton swab saturated with an antiseptic solution such as Listerine or hydrogen peroxide. The tooth should be checked once a month to assess how it is erupting. If a tooth is pushed back in the gums or falls out early due to trauma, the permanent tooth related to the affected tooth may not erupt properly. The baby teeth help the permanent teeth erupt in their normal positions.

Teeth are sometimes knocked out due to trauma. If the tooth is kept moist and the child is taken to a dentist within a half hour of the accident, the tooth may, in a small percentage of cases, be reimplanted. (See First Aid in Part Three.) When the tooth has been reimplanted, the pulp sometimes dies and root canal therapy or pulpotomy is necessary. A tooth will turn brown or blue if trauma has caused the death of the pulp. A dark yellow color indicates that the pulp has calcified. (This is not unique to children's teeth; the situation is the same in permanent teeth.) Sometimes, the root dissolves (resorbs) and eventually is lost.

If a child receives a blow to the lips, jaw, or face, cleanse any cuts with a clean washcloth, and apply pressure with gauze to stop the bleeding. If the bleeding or the cut is severe, or if there is a splinter in the wound, seek professional help immediately. Do not try to remove the splinter or you may push it in further. Antibiotics or a tetanus shot may be required. If the area is swollen, apply ice to it immediately. If there is severe pain in the jaw area, or if the bones feel as if they are uneven or pushed out abnormally, seek help immediately since a fracture may have occurred. Try to keep the jaw immobile—use a temporary head bandage (see page 109) if possible—until you reach a hospital or oral surgeon.

CONVENTIONAL TREATMENT

With any trauma to the mouth, it is best to consult with your dentist as soon as possible to determine if treatment is required. The dentist will probably examine the affected area and may take x-rays at that time, especially if the area is very painful or swollen. A soft diet may be recommended and the child may have to return for an examination after the swelling and pain have decreased.

If the fracture is on the tooth's enamel surface, smoothing any rough edges may be the only treatment necessary. If the trauma has caused a tooth to become loose, a splint can be used. The loose tooth is fastened to the splint by means of a wire attached to one or two teeth on each side. This will stabilize the tooth, allowing the bone and gums to heal. Baby teeth are not splinted; they heal automatically.

When the top portion of the pulp has been irreversibly damaged, but the damage does not extend into the tooth's canals, a pulpotomy is usually performed. In a pulpotomy, the infected pulp is removed. The area is next treated with formocresol, then filled with a paste of calcium hydroxide, which promotes healing, destroys bacteria, and, in some cases, unites the fractured area. A filling or stainless steel crown is placed over the area.

Pulpotomies are commonly performed on primary or newly erupted permanent teeth. New permanent teeth that have pulpotomies eventually require root canal therapy. Because these teeth have roots that have not yet developed, the pulpotomy stops the infection, while allowing the roots to continue developing. Once the permanent root ends have developed (which may take several years), root canal therapy is performed.

HOMEOPATHIC TREATMENT

Because of their alcohol base, liquid homeopathic preparations should not be given to children. Tablets, which have a sweet milk sugar base and can be dissolved in the mouth, are excellent for children. For infants, dissolve the tablet or pellet in water, and give it to the child in an eyedropper. (See Part One, Homeopathy, for additional information.)

Preparation	Directions for Use	Comments
Arnica 30X	Give 1 tablet 3 times daily.	Indicated for bruised mouth after trauma; helps promote healing.
Chamomilla 30X	Give 1 tablet hourly.	Recommended to calm a child who is restless or crying.
Hypericum 6X	Give 1 tablet 2 times daily.	To help heal nerves damaged by trauma.
Mercurius solubilis 30X	Give 1 tablet 2 times daily.	Recommended for infant who has sore gums and excessive salivation.
Rhus toxicodendron 30X	Give 2 tablets hourly.	Relieves pain of fractured or cracked teeth or jaw.
Symphytum 3X	Give 1 tablet 1 hour before bedtime.	Promotes sleep after injury.

HERBAL TREATMENT

Herb	Directions for Use	Comments
Clove oil	Place on a cotton-tipped swab and rub on teeth and gums.	Relieves pain of toothache.
Wintergreen	Prepare as tea (see Part Three, Using Herbs, Tea Preparation). Allow to cool and have child use as a mouthwash 2–3 times a day.	Has astringent and antiseptic properties.

RECOMMENDATIONS

■ After an accident involving your child's mouth, it is important to remain calm. As soon as possible, clean the area gently with a washcloth or gauze soaked in hydrogen peroxide. Stop any bleeding by applying pressure to the wound with gauze or a clean, soft washcloth.

■ It is a good idea to have your dentist check the area. If the trauma has caused severe cuts, the child's pediatrician should be consulted to see if stitches are required.

■ If the trauma is to the lips or in the mouth, give the child soft foods only to prevent further irritation.

■ If an infection is present in children under eight years old, avoid the antibiotic tetracycline. One of this drug's side effects includes severe, permanent discoloration of developing teeth. (If tetracycline has been used and discoloration does exist, cosmetic dentistry can be performed at a later age to treat the stains.)

■ When participating in contact sports such as football, hockey, and karate, children should wear an appropriate helmet and mouth guard. Mouth guards alone should be worn for basketball and soccer. A catcher's mask is a must for the catcher of a baseball game.

Trench Mouth

See Gum Disease.

Tumors

See Cysts and Tumors.

Vincent's Disease

See Gum Disease.

Wisdom-Teeth-Related Problems

Wisdom teeth, also called third molars, are the last molars on each side of both jaws. They usually erupt when a person is about twenty years of age.

Wisdom teeth may be pulled for a variety of reasons. In some cases they are impacted in such a way that it is impossible for them to erupt. This can be a source of frequent inflammation (pericoronitis) and pain. If wisdom teeth are coming in crooked, they may push on the surrounding teeth, causing pain and crowding. And because of their position in the back of the mouth, it may be difficult to reach these teeth for effective cleaning, and gum disease or cavities may ensue.

CONVENTIONAL TREATMENT

If wisdom teeth have erupted normally and are causing no pain or discomfort, they should not be pulled. The decision to pull wisdom teeth is based on such factors as the age and overall health of the person, the condition of the wisdom teeth, the presence or absence of other molars, and the position of the impacted wisdom teeth relative to other structures such as the sinuses or large nerves.

NUTRITIONAL SUPPLEMENTS

Supplement	Directions for Use	Comments
Calcium	Take 1500 mg daily.	Essential to health of bone and teeth.
Magnesium	Take 750 mg daily.	Works with calcium to maintain healthy bones and teeth.

HOMEOPATHIC TREATMENT

Dissolve the tablets under your tongue. Do not eat or drink for fifteen minutes prior to or after taking medication. (See Part One, Homeopathy, for additional information.)

Preparation	Directions for Use	Comments
Belladonna 30X	Take 1 tablet hourly as needed.	Indicated for pain relief.
Hepar sulphuris 6X	Take 3 tablets daily as needed.	Indicated for pain relief.
Hypericum 30X	Take 1 tablet twice daily as needed.	Indicated for pain relief.

HERBAL TREATMENT

Herb	Directions for Use	Comments
Alfalfa	Take 400 mg in capsule or tablet form daily.	Helps detoxify the blood.
Echinacea	Take 450 mg in capsule or tablet form every 2 hours. Decrease as needed.	Has antibiotic and anti-inflammatory properties.
Goldenseal	Take 400 mg in capsule or tablet form daily.	Strengthens immune system; has antibiotic and anti-inflammatory properties.
Horsetail	Take 400 mg in capsule or tablet form daily.	Accelerates healing of wounds.

RECOMMENDATIONS

■ If wisdom teeth have erupted normally and are causing no pain or discomfort, they should not be pulled.

■ *See also* Impacted Teeth in Part Two.

Xerostomia

See Dry Mouth.

X-Ray Exposure

Dental x-rays are an important diagnostic tool for early detection of tooth decay. X-rays can also be used to diagnose tooth and jaw problems, such as impacted teeth and bone fractures, that cannot be seen any other way.

Over the years there have been many improvements in the equipment used in obtaining x-rays. Along with high-speed film for limited exposure, devices to limit beam size, and precise timers for consistent exposures, manufacturers have attempted to limit the amount of radiation given off by their new equipment. However, since radiation in the body is cumulative, x-rays should be taken only when necessary. Excessive exposure to radiation may lead to damaging side effects.

A full set of x-rays (twelve to eighteen pictures) should not be taken more than once every three years. To minimize the risks of radiation, always wear a lead apron while x-rays are being taken. Be sure that your neck, the site of the sensitive thyroid, is covered. Many aprons now have a protective thyroid collar for this purpose. Nutritional supplements, herbs, and homeopathic preparations can also help protect you against the potentially damaging side effects of x-rays.

NUTRITIONAL SUPPLEMENTS

Supplement	Directions for Use	Comments
Beta-carotene	Take 2000 IU daily.	An antioxidant. Can help prevent cancer.
Calcium	Take 1500 mg daily.	Strengthens bone and protects against radiation poisoning.
Kelp	Take 500 mg daily.	High in trace minerals. Binds with toxins caused by radiation and eliminates them.
Magnesium	Take 750 mg daily.	Works with calcium to strengthen bones.
Vitamin C	Take 2000–6000 mg daily.	An antioxidant. Can help to prevent cancer. Helps promote the development of healthy tissues.

HOMEOPATHIC TREATMENT

Dissolve the tablets under your tongue. Do not eat or drink for fifteen minutes prior to or after taking medication. (See Part One, Homeopathy, for additional information.)

Preparation	Directions for Use	Comments
Calcarea fluorica 6X	Take 1 tablet 3 times on the day of exposure.	Helps prevent damage caused by extensive exposure to x-rays.
Mercurius solubilis 30X	Take 1 tablet 3 times on the day before and on the day after x-rays.	Helps minimize the hazards of x-rays.

HERBAL TREATMENT

Herb	Directions for Use	Comments
Alfalfa	Prepare as a tea (see Part Three, Using Herbs, Tea Preparation). Drink a cup 2–3 times on the day before the x-ray and for 3 days after the x-ray.	Helps to protect against radiation; is a strong blood purifier.
Red clover	Prepare as a tea (see Part Three, Using Herbs, Tea Preparation). Drink a cup 2–3 times on the day before the x-ray and for 3 days after the x-ray.	A strong blood purifier.

RECOMMENDATIONS

■ Pregnant women should avoid x-rays because of the high risk to the unborn child.

■ Make sure your dentist has the latest, most effective x-ray equipment, which minimizes radiation exposure. Find out when the equipment was last inspected according to government regulations. State law requirements vary.

■ When the use of x-rays is questionable, consider using a non-radiation technique such as computerized tomography (CAT scan). Unfortunately, equipment for such techniques is not readily available and is expensive to use. (For more information on types of x-rays, see X-Ray Techniques in Part Three.)

■ To minimize radiation exposure during x-rays, always wear a lead apron with a thyroid collar protector.

■ *See also* X-Ray Techniques in Part Three.

Yeast Infection (Candidiasis), Oral

Candidiasis is a general term for diseases produced by *Candida* species, which include a variety of fungi produced by "budding" and referred to as yeasts. The most common of these is called *Candida albicans*, which is normally found in varying amounts in the mouth, gastrointestinal tract, and vagina.

In the mouth, candidiasis is commonly referred to as thrush. Thrush is characterized by creamy to gray-colored patches that cover the tongue, cheek mucosa (inner lining of the cheek), palate, and throat. Efforts to remove the patches leave red areas that may bleed. Disease occurs when the yeast exhibits an unusual acceleration in growth, which occurs when the immune system is weakened and resistance is lowered. One of the early signs of AIDS is candidiasis of the mouth. Diabetes, malnutrition, old and loose-fitting dentures, poor oral hygiene, heavy smoking, anemia, and altered hormonal levels during pregnancy are other common contributing factors of candidiasis. Long-term use of antibiotics and immunosuppressive drugs, especially corticosteroids, disrupt the normal balance of oral bacteria, permitting *Candida albicans* to grow rapidly and produce a diseased state.

Candidiasis can be asymptomatic, or it can be accompanied by pain and a burning sensation. It is most common in the elderly and newborns. In the elderly, it is usually reported under dentures. In infants, it sometimes develops as the baby passes through the birth canal, especially if the mother has a vaginal yeast infection.

CONVENTIONAL TREATMENT

Nystatin (Mycostatin) liquid is usually prescribed; it is swished in the mouth for two minutes and then swallowed. Nystatin tablets (100,000 units) and clotrimazole (Mycelex) in 10-mg doses may be prescribed as lozenges. Regardless of which treatment is prescribed, it should be continued for at least fourteen days and until laboratory tests are negative. Treatment may take four to six weeks, or even longer if the infection is tenacious.

Liquid nystatin may cause nausea and discomfort for individuals with dry, sensitive mucosa in the mouth. In this case, the antifungal drugs ketoconazole (Nizoral 200-mg tablets) and amphotericin B may be prescribed, because they are better tolerated. Long-term use of these products may, however, weaken the immune system. Nystatin may cause damage to liver function if used for long periods; it may also weaken the immune system, lowering resistance to disease.

NUTRITIONAL SUPPLEMENTS

Supplement	Directions for Use	Comments
Acidophilus	Take capsules as directed on the label.	Helps balance the normal ecology of the body.
Garlic	Take two 250-mg tablets 3 times daily.	Natural antibiotic; strengthens the immune system.
Vitamin A	Take 20,000 IU daily.	Important antioxidant; helps heal tissues in the mouth.
Vitamin C	Take 2000 mg daily.	Helps enhance healing of tissues made sore by candida patches.

HOMEOPATHIC TREATMENT

Dissolve the tablets under your tongue. Do not eat or drink for fifteen minutes prior to or after taking medication. (See Part One, Homeopathy, for additional information.)

Preparation	Directions for Use	Comments
Antimonium tartaricum 6X	Take 1 tablet daily.	Helps heal sores caused by candida.
Borax 30X	Take 1 tablet 3 times daily.	Indicated for treatment of thrush.
Kali muriaticum 6X	Take 1 tablet hourly.	Helps destroy candida.

HERBAL TREATMENT

Herb	Directions for Use	Comments
Alfalfa	Prepare as a tea (see Part Three, Using Herbs, Tea Preparation). Drink 2–3 cups daily until infection clears.	Excellent blood purifier.
Burdock root	Prepare as a tea (see Part Three, Using Herbs, Tea Preparation). Drink 2–3 cups daily.	Excellent blood purifier.
Red clover and alfalfa	Prepare together as a tea (see Part Three, Using Herbs, Tea Preparation). Drink 2–3 cups daily.	Helps eradicate destructive drugs in the body.
Sanicle	Prepare as a mouthwash (see Part Three, Using Herbs, Mouthwash Preparation). Use as needed.	Helpful as a detoxifier.
Sarsaparilla root	Prepare as a tea (see Part Three, Using Herbs, Tea Preparation), and drink 2–3 cups daily. Prepare as a mouthwash (see Part Three, Using Herbs, Mouthwash Preparation) and use as needed.	Helpful as a detoxifier.

RECOMMENDATIONS

■ Avoid eating foods that ferment (e.g., cheeses, dried fruits, and acidic fruits such as grapefruit, lemons, tomatoes, pineapples, and oranges). Spicy foods, all sugars including honey, caffeine, chocolate, and dairy products should also be avoided. Eat at least one cup of yogurt or kefir daily. Drink plenty of water. Avoid tobacco, alcohol, and mouthwashes containing alcohol.

■ Discontinue use of antibiotics, corticosteroids, and oral contraceptives during treatment.

■ Research indicates that high levels of mercury in the body may contribute to candidiasis. Hair analysis may be useful to determine if this is the case. If the mercury is at toxic levels, it is important to ascertain the source.

■ Practice good oral hygiene. Change toothbrushes monthly, and discard your toothbrush after completing treatment for candidiasis.

■ Have ill-fitting dentures corrected.

■ Exercise regularly and get enough sleep.

■ During treatment, do not use any products that contain yeast.

■ Use Orithrush from Cardiovascular Research as a mouthwash. It helps destroy candida.

■ *The Yeast Syndrome* by Drs. John Parks Trowbridge and Morton Walker (New York: Bantam Books) is an excellent reference for further information on candidiasis.

Part Three

Dental Techniques

Introduction

Knowledge is a powerful tool. Armed with it, you can cure the ill, soothe the fearful, overcome obstacles, and safeguard your well-being. In Part Three, you will learn to use and/or understand many of the tools, techniques, and procedures involved in dentistry.

Information in Part Three teaches you how to prepare herbal remedies that can help cure specific dental disorders discussed in Part Two. You will also learn, for example, the exact procedures for root canal therapy, tooth extractions, and certain gum surgeries. Knowledge of these procedures will help soothe any fears you may have about undergoing treatment. Orthodontic techniques used to correct tooth and jaw irregularities are also discussed. If you are still a bit anxious, there is a section on Pain and Stress Management, which should help. But once you master the section on oral hygiene techniques, you may never have to visit a dentist except for routine check-ups and cleanings!

Acupressure

For thousands of years, the Chinese have used acupuncture to relieve pain and treat various diseases. The Chinese believe that disease and pain occur due to an imbalance in the energy flow along certain channels (meridians) in the body. In acupuncture, needles are inserted into specific points along the meridians to restore balance and, in turn, health. Acupressure follows the same principle, except that gentle pressure, rather than needles, is applied to the specific points.

Modern researchers believe that stimulating the specific points by using needles or pressure probably stimulates the brain to release endorphins. Endorphins

are chemical substances that act on the nervous system to reduce awareness of pain. They produce effects similar to those of morphine. Another possibility is that acupuncture and acupressure work by triggering signals from the nervous system that interrupt pain messages received by the brain.

By applying gentle pressure to the appropriate points, a skilled practitioner can help alleviate pain and muscle tension. A high degree of medical knowledge is not required to successfully practice acupressure. This technique has no side effects, and it can be used while you are being treated with medications. You can treat yourself or others by identifying various acupressure points. The acupressure points associated with mouth pain and related disorders are illustrated in Figure 3.1.

For self-treatment, sit or lie in a place where you will

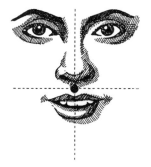

To relieve toothache, use forefinger to apply strong pressure to point indicated for three minutes.

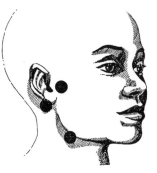

To relieve jaw pain, apply light pressure to each point for three minutes.

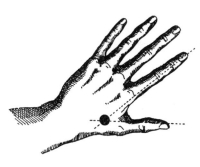

To relieve pain in teeth or face, apply light circular pressure to point indicated as needed.

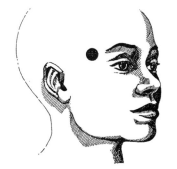

To relieve headache, use forefinger to apply light pressure to point indicated for three minutes.

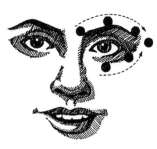

To relieve headache and pain behind eyes, apply light circular pressure to points around eye in direction indicated.

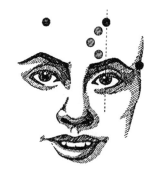

To relieve headache, apply light circular pressure to points indicated as needed.

Figure 3.1 Acupressure Points

167

not be disturbed by the telephone or other distractions. To find the right acupressure point, apply firm pressure to the area shown on the illustrations in Figure 3.1. If you are applying pressure to the correct point, you will begin to feel some pain in the area of that point. For pain that is acute (of short duration), lightly massage the acupressure point using a circular motion. Use the pads of the fingers or thumb, and continue to massage from one to five minutes. For chronic pain, (pain that has been present for a long time), apply medium pressure.

Anesthesia

Prior to the use of anesthesia, herbs, wine, vinegar, and some gases were used for pain control during certain dental procedures. The discovery of anesthetics has made it possible for the dentist to provide treatment with confidence, knowing the patient is comfortable and free from pain.

In 1884, pioneer surgeon William S. Halsted injected cocaine into the inferior alveolar nerve (located along the length of the lower jaw) before performing a dental procedure. Since then, many forms of local anesthesia have been discovered.

There are two main categories of anesthetics: local and general. Local anesthesia prevents nerve impulses from being transmitted to the brain via a chemical agent and, as a result, brings about loss of feeling to a localized area. During local anesthesia, the patient is awake and aware. Almost all dental treatments can be performed with a local anesthetic; however, there are certain cases in which a general anesthetic is used. General anesthesia, which causes the patient to lose consciousness, is usually reserved for orthognatic surgeries (those involving facial bones, cleft lips and palates, and advanced temporomadibular jaw disorders). General anesthesia is also commonly used for some oral surgeries, including the extractions of impacted wisdom teeth.

The use of general anesthesia is serious. There are risks involved with the drugs used—respiratory and/or cardiac failure, or allergic reactions. Procedures requiring general anesthetics should be performed in a hospital, surgical clinic, or office where proper life-support equipment and qualified personnel are available in case of an emergency. Prior to giving general anesthesia, the patient will be given strict instructions regarding intake of food and liquid before and after the procedure. It is critical to follow these instructions.

Local anesthesia, when given properly, poses very little or no adverse side effects. Xylocaine (lidocaine) and Carbocaine (mepivacaine) are the most common local anesthetics used by dentists. Xylocaine comes with or without epinephrine, which is a vasoconstrictor. Vasoconstrictors are important components of most anesthetics because they limit the flow of blood to the area. This keeps the area numb longer and also helps restrict bleeding. If the anesthetic has epinephrine and is injected too quickly, a rapid heartbeat and flushing may occur for a few minutes. Although some allergic reactions have been reported from Xylocaine, it has an excellent safety record. Carbocaine, which has no epinephrine, is as fast and effective as Xylocaine. Because it has no epinephrine, many doctors recommend it for those with high blood pressure, heart problems, or diabetes.

Although local anesthetics rarely pose adverse side effects, their potential for toxicity does exist if too much is administered. Overdosage is rare, but signs to watch for are headache, drowsiness, nausea, disorientation, restlessness, visual disturbances, flushed skin, and uncontrollable muscle twitching. Because local anesthetics may cause the lip, cheek, and tongue to become numb, it is important not to bite these areas. This will cause trauma and pain that will be noticed when the anesthetic wears off.

Allergic reactions to the preservatives in local anesthetics may occur. The preservative most commonly used is methylparaben, which acts as an antiseptic. For those who are allergic to methyparaben, a red rash may appear at the injection site. Further allergic reactions may include restlessness, anxiety, and increased blood pressure, pulse, and respiratory rate. Although it is rare, death can occur with extremely high doses, or as a reaction to the person's medical condition or to drugs he or she may be taking. Therefore, individuals with a known allergy to methylparaben must be sure to let the dentist know.

During pregnancy, it is best not to receive any dental injections unless absolutely necessary. Local anesthetics have been known to slow down the heart rate of embryos. If you are pregnant, be sure to check with your doctor before any anesthetic is administered.

There are three techniques for giving local injections—block, field, and topical. During the block technique, generally done in the lower jaw, the nerve trunk that lies along a section of the mouth is anesthetized. Block anesthesia numbs the lower side of the jaw, as well as part of the lip, tongue, and cheek. The field technique, usually performed on the upper teeth, is used to anesthetize a specific area of tissue or a particular tooth. Field injections are given directly in the gum area that is to be treated. Topical anesthetics, usually in ointment, spray, or liquid form, are used in the third type of application technique. The anesthetic is applied to the injection site to mildly anesthetize the area before the injection. People with a sensitive gag reflex that is triggered when taking x-rays or when impressions or molds have to be taken can benefit from a topical anesthetic, which temporarily numbs the tongue and roof of the mouth. In some cases, topical anesthetics are used to mildly numb the gums and teeth before a cleaning.

What about the "pain" from the injection itself? If this is a problem for you, know that there are a number of things that both you and your dentist can do to eliminate or reduce this pain. You can, for example, use relaxation techniques to reduce the anxiety of anticipated pain (detailed information on relaxation techniques is provided in Stress and Anxiety Management in Part Three.) Or you can listen to music through stereo headphones, which provides a pleasant distraction from the injection as well as the procedure itself. There are a number of things the dentist can do to alleviate the pain from a needle. For instance, he or she can apply a topical anesthetic to mildly numb the area before the injection. Dentists commonly use techniques, such as shaking the cheek or applying finger-pressure to the area of injection, to distract the patient from the pinch of the needle. An anesthetic solution that has been warmed to body temperature seems to make the injection less noticeable. Some dentists have special warmers for this purpose (although simply running the anesthetic vial under warm water for a few minutes is just as effective).

In addition to local and general anesthetics, gases, such as nitrous oxide (laughing gas) are also used in dentistry. Nitrous oxide, which can be used along with local anesthesia, is administered with a nose mask and given in combination with oxygen. Nitrous oxide renders the patient totally unconcerned during treatment. Pain sensation is not eliminated, but the anxiety of the treatment is. When nitrous oxide is first administered, there is an immediate feeling of relaxation, warmth, tingling or numbness, visual changes, slurred speech, and slowed responses. These effects are temporary, with the patient returning to normal as soon as the gas is turned off. High doses of nitrous oxide can cause side effects that include nausea, vomiting, and excitability in some children after a few minutes exposure to the gas. Pregnant women as well as individuals with blocked nasal passages due to a cold, heart or respiratory problems, or psychiatric prob-

lems should not use this gas. Anesthetics used for dental procedures are safe and reliable when used properly.

Along with their benefits, however, all medications have inherent risks. A disclosure of your complete health history to the dentist is important for safe and proper use of anesthetics.

RECOMMENDATIONS

■ Unless it is absolutely necessary, always opt for local anesthesia over general, which has a number of inherent risks.

■ Calcium and vitamin C should be avoided on the day of dental treatment since these supplements may decrease the effectiveness of the anesthetic.

■ For routine dental procedures, it is best to learn how to manage anxiety and fear, and to receive only local anesthetics.

■ Do not be concerned if you experience a rapid heartbeat and a flush sensation after receiving a local anesthetic. This reaction is usually caused by the accidental injection of the anesthetic into a blood vessel. The sensation is temporary.

■ Certain local anesthetics that contain epinephrine may be inadvisable to use (or used with caution) by those with high blood pressure, heart problems, or diabetes.

■ If general anesthesia is administered in a dental office, the proper equipment and personnel must be available to handle emergencies.

■ As with any medical procedure, be sure to disclose your complete medical history, including any known allergies. Inform the dentist of any medications you may be taking.

Anxiety Management

See Stress and Anxiety Management.

Bonding and Bleaching

See Cosmetic Dentistry.

Chelation Therapy

When a dentist suspects heavy metal toxicity due to dental materials such as mercury, nickel, tin, or lead, chelation (pronounced key-lay-shun) therapy may be recommended. Specific chelating agents bind with the heavy toxic metals, helping to remove them from the body. Metal molecules have one or more positively charged subatomic particles. The negative charge of the chelating substance enables it to combine with and hold on to the positive charges of the metal—much as opposite poles of magnets attract and hold each other. For more than forty years, chelation therapy has been used in the United States to treat and prevent hardening of the arteries (arteriosclerosis). Chelation therapy is also used for treatment of other circulatory problems.

Chelating agents can be administered either orally or intravenously. Injections usually consist of EDTA (ethylene diamine tetraacetic acid), a synthetic amino acid. EDTA is a strong agent that is slowly released into the blood stream and binds most metals. It should be administered only by qualified physicians, those certified by the American Board of Chelation Therapy (ABCT). Over-the-counter preparations, such as alfalfa, selenium, chromium, garlic extract (such as Kyolic Aged Garlic Extract), coenzyme Q-10, iron, copper, and zinc, are also helpful. Most serious illnesses require intravenous therapy.

Recommended Chelating Agents

Agent	Directions for Use	Comments
Alfalfa	Take 250 mg 3 times daily.	Chelates toxic substances and neutralizes body chemistry.
Coenzyme Q-10	Take 100 mg daily.	Improves circulation and heart function.
EDTA	Take 3000-4000 gm daily.	Administered by intravenous injection. Improves circulation and removes toxic substances.
Garlic	Take two 250-mg tablets daily.	Chelates and detoxifies.
Selenium	Take 200 mcg daily.	Acts as an antioxidant by removing free radicals.
Vitamin C with bioflavonoids	Take 6000 mg daily. May be given orally or, at a higher dose, intravenously.	Chelating agent for heavy metals, improves immune-system function.
Vitamin E	Take 600 IU daily.	Scavenger of free radicals and other toxic substances.

Cosmetic Dentistry

The appearance of your teeth has a major effect on your self-confidence. In many occupations—sales, modeling, public relations, entertainment—the appearance of your teeth may affect your job. And even if your career is not a factor, teeth that look good can help make you feel good.

In recent years, new materials and techniques have allowed miraculous improvements in just about every area of dental aesthetics. Cosmetic dental techniques can improve teeth that are stained, cracked, crooked, or unevenly spaced. To correct stains, bleaching and bonding are the two most popular techniques used. Bonding is also performed to reshape teeth that are malformed.

BLEACHING

Bleaching is performed to lighten teeth. Tooth-bleaching gel contains oxygen-releasing chemicals (e.g., hydrogen peroxide) that oxydize the stain out. If a few teeth are stained, the dentist will bleach them in the office. If all of the teeth are stained, the dentist will give the patient a bleaching kit with instructions for bleaching the teeth at home.

To bleach teeth in the office, the dentist first applies the gel to the tooth enamel, leaves it on for about thirty minutes, then rinses it off. To achieve the desired whiteness, this procedure may have to be repeated over several visits. Temporary sensitivity may be experienced after bleaching the teeth. If, however, the teeth become too sensitive while the dentist is applying the gel, rinse off the gel immediately.

If all of the teeth are to be bleached, a custom tray is made to cover the upper and/or lower teeth. At home, the patient places the gel in the tray then presses the tray over the stained teeth, where it is left in the mouth overnight. Depending on the degree of stain, it may take many days of treatment before the teeth reach the desired whiteness. Some sensitivity may be experienced with this form of bleaching. Certain kits cause less sensitivity that others; some cause none at all. Kits containing 10 percent carbamide peroxide have been shown to cause very little sensitivity.

A few state-of-the-art brands offered at dental offices include Opalescence, Lighten, and White and Bright. Over-the-counter bleaching kits, which contain diluted acids or teeth whiteners, are also available. However, it has not been proven that these over-the-counter whiteners actually work. Furthermore, using these products may cause gums to peel or have a blanched, whitish appearance. As a result, the Food and Drug Administration has taken many of these products off the market.

BONDING

Composite resins, applied to teeth in a procedure called bonding, can camouflage stained teeth and recontour misshapen teeth. This material, which comes in a variety of tooth-colored shades, is also used to fill cavities (see Filling a Cavity in Part Three).

Several bonding techniques are available. In one common technique, first, the front of the stained tooth is slightly reduced (to prevent bulkiness when the composite material is applied). Next, microscopic grooves are etched into the tooth surface with a solution of 30 to 70 percent phosphoric acid or 1 percent hydrochloric acid. This procedure, known as acid-etching, can be done only on enamel. The acid will cause sensitivity if placed on dentin. A liquid-plastic bonding agent that consists of methyl methacrylate, diacrylate, glycidyl methacrylate, or another adhesive is applied to the tooth, which is next covered by a tooth-colored composite. The composite is then carved and contoured while it is still soft. To harden the composite, often a low-voltage tungsten-halogen lamp is focused on the area for approximately thirty to sixty seconds. Some composites self-cure and harden without the use of the light.

Laminated veneers are used in another common bonding technique. In much the same way that a false fingernail is contoured and cemented onto an existing nail, a composite or porcelain veneer is shaped and bonded to an existing tooth. Veneers are most effective for front teeth that are chipped, stained, eroded, or poorly shaped. They can also be used to close gaps between the front teeth. The porcelain veneer is the strongest one available. Composite veneers crack and chip more easliy than the porcelain; they also tend to stain.

When a porcelain or composite veneer is made, a thin layer of enamel is first removed from the surface of the tooth. For a porcelain veneer, first, an impression is taken of the tooth, and a model is made from the impression. The laboratory then fabricates the veneer to fit the model and sends it back to the dentist. On a subsequent visit, the veneer is bonded to the tooth using the same technique employed with composite fillings. A composite veneer can be completed in only one visit. Once the outer surface of enamel is drilled from the tooth, the tooth is acid-etched, covered with a bonding adhesive, and covered with the composite veneer.

For more information on the aesthetic repair of damaged or missing teeth, see Filling a Cavity; and Prosthodontic Techniques in Part Three.

Emergency Treatment

See First Aid.

Endodontic Techniques

Endodontics is the branch of dentistry that deals with diseases of the tooth root, dental pulp, and the surrounding tissue. Endodontic procedures include root canal therapy, apicoectomy, pulp-capping, and pulpotomy. For more information on surgical guidelines, see Surgery in Part Three.

ROOT CANAL THERAPY

Compare the two teeth shown in Figure 3.2. One tooth is healthy, while the other has decay in the pulp chamber. When the pulp tissue containing the nerve and blood vessels is damaged beyond repair, root canal therapy is performed. This therapy requires two or more visits to the dentist. Before the treatment begins,

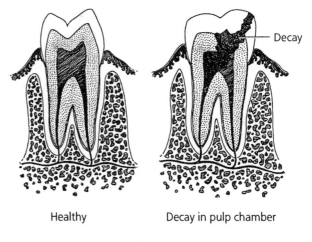

Healthy   Decay in pulp chamber

Figure 3.2. Healthy and Decayed Tooth

local anesthetic is given and the tooth is isolated by a rubber dam.

The first step of the three-step root canal treatment is called a *pulpectomy*. During this step, the pulp is removed from the chamber and the canal or canals. Access to the pulp chamber is achieved by drilling a small opening through the enamel and dentin. To clean out the small, fine canals that contain the nerve and blood vessels, small endodontic files as seen in Figure 3.3 are used. These delicate files vary in width and depth, and the dentist uses particular files based on the size of the canal. Antiseptic solutions such as sodium hypochlorite (bleach) or hydrogen peroxide are used to irrigate the pulp canals periodically, while the files are used to clean the canals as seen in Figure 3.4. A small cotton pellet is saturated with eugenol or formocreosol and placed in the canal opening, which is then sealed with a temporary filling. (This cotton will be removed during the next visit.) If there is an infection in the tooth, your dentist may prescribe antibiotics and pain medications. The pulpectomy is completed in one visit.

During the second visit, the canal or canals are prepared to be filled. The files and antiseptic solutions are used repeatedly to clean, shape, and smooth the canals. The canals are dried with paper points, tapered material that comes in different widths and is shaped like the canal as shown in Figure 3.5. If the dentist determines that the canals are sufficiently clean, they may be filled during this visit. If blood and debris are still noticed in the canals, the dentist will not fill them until the third visit.

Once the dentist concludes that the canals are ready to be filled, a tapered, rubbery filling material called gutta-percha is inserted into one of the canals. An x-ray is taken to determine if the size of the gutta-percha is right. The gutta-percha is then coated with a special cement and pressed against the canal walls. This process continues until all of the canals are filled and sealed with gutta-percha.

After the root canal procedure, a crown is usually placed over the remaining tooth. Before placing the crown, the dentist may decide to further strengthen the tooth by inserting a post. A post, which is either a pin or a screw, is usually required if the natural crown portion of the tooth is badly damaged. To place the post, the dentist drills a tapered hole into one of the canals that has been filled with gutta-percha. The tapered hole must be deep but not the full extent of the canal. The pin or screw is then cemented into the hole, over which the dentist places amalgam or composite as a bulk build-up for the artificial crown.

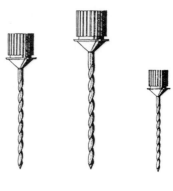

Figure 3.3. Endodontic Files

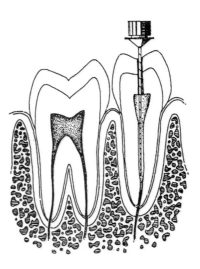

Figure 3.4. Tooth with Endodontic File

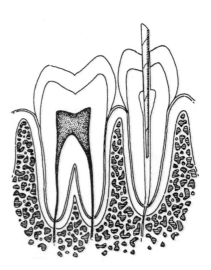

Figure 3.5. Tooth with Paper Point

APICOECTOMY

Once root canal therapy is completed on a tooth, there should no longer be pain. Sometimes, however, reinfections occur. Pain may be experienced years after the root canal treatment is completed, and an x-ray may reveal an abscess. At this point, the treatment most often rendered is an apicoectomy. During an apicoectomy, the end of the tooth's root is amputated and the area is cleaned of any debris or infection. The open end of the root is then sealed with an amalgam or composite filling. Once root canal therapy fails because of reinfection, and abscess and pain are present, pulling the tooth may be a more suitable choice of treatment.

If root canal therapy does not thoroughly seal the apex or end of the root opening, a "window" is cut through the gum and bone over the apex of the root. Once the root apex is visible, infected tissue is cleaned out, and the canal is cut until clean root is visible. The area is sealed with amalgam and the gum is sutured back in position.

PULP-CAPPING

If decay reaches the nerve area, but the nerve and blood vessels don't seem damaged beyond repair, the dentist may decide to perform a pulp-capping procedure instead of root canal therapy. In pulp-capping, a layer of calcium hydroxide, which stimulates dentin formation, is placed over the exposed pulp. A mixture of zinc oxide and eugenol is placed over the calcium hydroxide. The dentist may leave this sedative material over the exposed nerve for several weeks. If the nerve is not damaged irreversibly, new dentin will form over the exposed pulp and a permanent filling will be placed over that. If the pulp is damaged beyond repair, no dentin will form, pain will increase, and the dentist will have to perform root canal therapy.

PULPOTOMY

Sometimes the pulp is damaged but not dead. The dentist may then decide to remove the pulp chamber, but leave the pulp in the canal or canals. During this procedure, known as pulpotomy, the pulp chamber is cleaned out, and a mixture of zinc oxide and eugenol is packed in the area. Pulpotomies are performed primarily on recently erupted teeth in which the roots have not completely formed. The pulpotomy allows the roots to develop undisturbed.

Equilibration

Sometimes, if the teeth from the upper and lower jaws do not properly interdigitate or mesh together, an imbalance occurs. This imbalance can cause teeth to become loose, and contribute to gum disease and temporomandibular joint disorders. The dentist may choose to balance the bite with a technique called equilibration or occlusal therapy.

The dentist has the patient bite on a strip of blue- or red-coated articulating paper and simulate chewing. Marks then appear on the teeth indicating where they are making contact with each other. A drill is used to grind and smooth selected areas that are too high or not making proper contact with the opposing teeth. Either a few or many teeth may require this procedure, which is usually performed over several visits to the dentist.

If the bite is severely imbalanced, the dentist may make study models of the mouth by making a mold. Then the dentist will balance the teeth on the model before performing equilibration on the teeth.

Extraction, Tooth

See Tooth Extraction.

Filling a Cavity

Your dentist relies on visual examination and x-rays to detect cavities. During a routine examination, the dentist will use a small mirror to check all of the surfaces of each tooth. Anything that appears to deviate from normal will then be closely checked with the explorers, shown in Figure 3.6, and noted in your chart. The dentist may then x-ray your entire mouth or sections of it. The type of treatment your dentist chooses will depend on the extent of damage caused by decay.

If the decayed area is very slight and is on the outer surface of the enamel, treatment may not be suggested. In this case, the dentist will indicate the presence of dam-

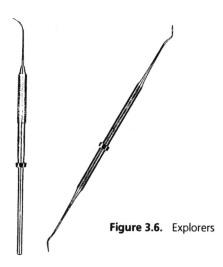

Figure 3.6. Explorers

age on your chart and check the tooth on return visits. If the decay has reached beyond the outer surface of enamel but not into the dentin, the dentist may or may not decide to treat it. More than likely, the decayed area will be cleaned and filled with any of a variety of filling materials such as amalgam, composite resins, or gold. Once the decay has reached the dentin, treatment is necessary to prevent the decay from reaching the pulp.

If the decay has not damaged the tooth extensively, the decay is removed and a filling is inserted. If the decay has damaged a large portion of the tooth, an artificial crown may be suggested. If the decay has reached the nerve, the dentist has two choices in treatment. He may decide that the nerve is irreversibly damaged and that root canal therapy is necessary (see page 171), or he may attempt to keep the nerve alive with a procedure called pulp-capping (see page 173).

FILLING MATERIALS

Materials used to fill cavities include composite resins, porcelain, amalgam, and gold. The filling material used often depends on the size and location of the cavity.

Composite (plastic) resins are the same color as teeth and are, therefore, aesthetically preferable as filling materials. They are usually used to fill cavities in front teeth and small cavities in back teeth. These composites are made of two materials: a plastic resin and a filler made of finely ground glass-like particles. The ingredients are mixed and placed in the cavity, where they harden. Composite fillings last from three to ten years. Be aware that the larger the area needing to be filled, the weaker these materials become. Composite filling materials may chip, wear with chewing, and become stained or discolored from coffee, tea, or tobacco. In

addition, composites have been shown to "leak" at the edges; they also tend to pull away from the tooth, allowing new cavities to form. Proper home care and regular professional cleanings will help composites retain their original shade longer. Composites may also cause some sensitivity when used for deep fillings, unless a glass ionomer (an insulating material) is placed underneath the composite. Glass ionomers help protect the tooth against temperature changes and the pressure from chewing. Some irritation and sensitivity in the pulp chamber is a common temporary reaction after the placing of a composite filling. This reaction typically calms down within thirty days.

Porcelain fillings (called porcelain inlays), which are made of a ceramic material, are produced to order in a laboratory and then bonded to the tooth. (See Figure 3.7.) Porcelain inlays are aesthetically appealing since they can be matched to the color of the teeth and they resist staining. And unlike composite materials, they resist leaking. However, because they are brittle, they may fracture easily. It requires two visits to the dentist to obtain a porcelain inlay, and since they are custom made by a laboratory, their cost is similar to the cost of gold inlays.

Amalgam or silver fillings are actually a mixture of metals including silver, nickel, copper, and mercury. An amalgam filling is more resistant to wear than a composite or porcelain filling. However, due to its dark color, it is very conspicuous and not very pleasing aesthetically. Over time, it leaches into the surrounding enamel, giving it a gray color. There is also some question about possible health risks associated with these fillings. (See Mercury Toxicity in Part Two for more information.)

Gold inlays, which are cemented in place, are made

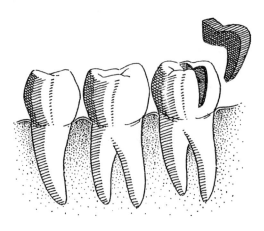

Figure 3.7. Inlay

in a laboratory. A gold inlay is well-tolerated by the gum tissues, and may last more than twenty years. If you are not allergic to gold, it is ultimately the best filling material. However, gold may be the most expensive of the choices.

First Aid

Emergencies occur at the most inappropriate times. It's the weekend; you are attending an important event and your bridge falls out. You are in the middle of eating dinner; a tooth breaks off a denture when you take a bite. It's midnight; it's been four hours since your tooth was pulled and it still won't stop bleeding. You are sound asleep in the middle of the night; a severe toothache wakes you. And the list goes on.

The following table is provided to give you easy access to first aid measures for common dental emergencies. If possible, seek dental care immediately. The methods listed should be used only until you can see your dentist.

FIRST AID FOR COMMON DENTAL EMERGENCIES

Emergency	First Aid Measure
Abscess	If an abscess has a pimple-like swelling at the tip, rinsing with warm salt water will cause it to form a head, which will eventually release pus. Over-the-counter ointments and aloe vera gel may help relieve symptoms such as pain and burning. Do not use over-the-counter steroid ointments since these may cause infections to spread.
Bitten tongue or cheek, or cuts inside the mouth	Bleeding can be stopped by applying pressure to the area with gauze and ice. Avoid using numbing ointments on the tongue, or you may accidentally bite it again.
Bleeding after tooth extraction	Some bleeding up to an hour after tooth extraction is normal. If bleeding does not stop, or stops and starts again, place a wet tea bag over the area. The tannic acid in the tea enhances clot formation. Biting down gently on a gauze pad will also help stop bleeding.
Bridge or crown falls out	Over-the-counter products sold in drug stores can be used to temporarily cement bridges and crowns. If you wear a bridge or a crown, keep one of these products in your medicine cabinet.
Broken denture	Products such as Quick Fix and Plate-Weld are available at drug stores and may be used for temporary repair of the denture. Follow the instructions on the package.

Emergency	First Aid Measure
Broken jaw	If you find that you cannot move your mouth and there is severe pain, try not to move your jaw and seek help immediately. If medical care is not immediately available, wrap a temporary bandage around your head as shown in the figure on page 109.
Broken orthodontic appliance	If a broken orthodontic appliance is bent or sharp, try to gently bend the wire back, but be careful as the wire may break. If the appliance is irritating to the gums, place a piece of wax or chewed sugarless gum on the broken area until you see your orthodontist.
Cracked tooth	Avoid chewing with the cracked tooth, and avoid foods or liquids that are very hot or cold. If you are in pain, take an over-the-counter pain reliever such as Tylenol or Advil. If possible, keep any tooth part that is broken, especially if it is a gold or porcelain filling, which may be recemented.
Cuts and lacerations	Apply pressure with gauze to stop the bleeding. Clean the wound unless a splinter or other object is imbedded in the area. In this case, wait and see a professional.
Dislocated jaw	If your jaw becomes dislocated and you are not able to close your mouth, stay calm. Gently try to work the jaw loose by moving it from side to side. If you try to force it, you may experience more pain. Seek professional help to determine the cause.
Knocked-out teeth	Knocked-out teeth may be replaced successfully if done within 30 minutes of the tooth's falling out. Never hold the tooth by the root. Rinse any dirt or blood off the tooth with cold water, replace it in the socket, and get to the dentist immediately. If you cannot see the dentist in less than 30 minutes, keep the tooth wrapped in a moist cloth or gauze, place it in a container of milk, or leave it under your tongue until you are treated.
Lost filling	Over-the-counter products are available to temporarily plug any holes left by lost fillings until you see the dentist. You can also make your own temporary filling by mixing 1 tablespoon of powdered goldenseal with $\frac{1}{2}$ teaspoon of warm water until a smooth paste is formed; add 1 drop of clove oil and mix till smooth. Place mixture in the hole with a rounded toothpick or the wooden end of a cotton-tipped swab.
Mouth sores	Most mouth sores will heal by themselves; however, over-the-counter ointments and aloe vera gel may help relieve symptoms such as pain and burning. Do not use over-the-counter steroid ointments since these may cause infection to spread.

Emergency	First Aid Measure
Swelling and pain over erupting wisdom teeth	Sometimes pain and inflammation accompany an erupting or impacted wisdom tooth. Called pericoronitis, the condition is often caused by food and other particles caught in hard-to-clean areas. Warm salt water rinses may reduce irritation and pain. A paste made of ½ teaspoon of baking soda, ½ teaspoon of goldenseal, and 1 teaspoon of aloe vera gel may also be helpful when placed over the area. Do not rub aspirin or other analgesics on the area; these may cause chemical burns. An ice cube placed over the area may help decrease pain. Avoid hard, spicy foods. Ointments made for the relief of toothaches may be helpful.
Swollen face and lip due to trauma	Place ice on area in 5 to15 minute intervals. Repeat several times. The next day, apply moist heat to the area.
Toothache	Over-the-counter products containing lidocaine or benzocaine can be used to provide temporary relief from toothache. Pain relievers such as Tylenol are helpful. Do not rub aspirin or other analgesics on the gums; these contain strong acids, and may cause burns on the gum tissues. A small piece of cotton saturated with clove oil or wintergreen and placed on the tooth will give temporary relief. Avoid sweets and hot and cold foods.

EMERGENCY DENTAL-CARE KIT

The following items should be kept together and readily accessible in case of a dental emergency:

- Baking soda, aloe vera gel, and salt to prepare astringent, soothing rinse.
- Ice pack for swelling and fractures.
- Tylenol, Advil, or other over-the-counter analgesic.
- Ointments such as Anbesol, Campho-Phenique, or Orajel for temporary toothache relief.
- Sterile gauze for control of bleeding.
- If you have braces, wax from the orthodontist.
- Temporary cements for loose bridges and crowns.

Fluoride Treatment

Fluoride treatments may be initiated at a child's first dental visit at the age of three. After the teeth are cleaned thoroughly, a fluoride gel is applied to the teeth with cotton-tipped applicators or placed in a mouth tray and pressed against the top and bottom teeth. Usually, the gel is left in the mouth for one to four minutes. Your child will be told not to drink or eat for half an hour after the fluoride treatment. The treatment is repeated at each six-month-check-up visit until the child reaches adolescence.

Gum Surgery

Just before gum surgery, the periodontist usually scrapes the plaque and tartar off the surface of the teeth with a scaler (see Figure 3.8). Gum or periodontal surgery is then performed by a periodontist using local anesthetic.

There are several different forms of gum surgery. *Gingivectomy* reduces the depth of gum pockets that harbor bacteria and cause bone loss. The depth of the pockets is measured with a periodontal probe (see Figure 3.9). One end of the probe has bands that indicate millimeters. This end is placed gently between the tooth and gum to measure gum pocket depth. After local anesthesia is administered, the gums are literally cut back to the normal depth of the pocket, usually two to three millimeters. After healing, normal pocket depth exists, allowing better access for proper cleaning and flossing.

Two forms of grafting or rebuilding may be performed by the periodontist—bone and gingival. *Bone grafts* are used on areas where the bone has been lost. The bone may be obtained from the jawbones or other

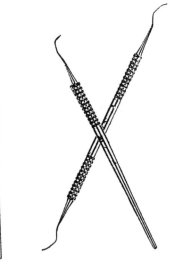

Figure 3.8. Scalers.

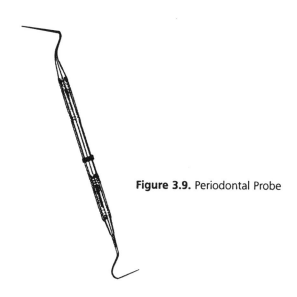

Figure 3.9. Periodontal Probe

parts of the body, or artificial bone may be used. The gums are surgically opened and the bone is placed in the area where it is needed. The gums are sutured back in place, and, in time, the new bone bonds with the existing bone. New gum tissue helps connect the bone to the tooth, strengthening loose teeth.

Gingival graft involves the replacement of lost or diseased gum tissue. Replacement gum tissue usually comes from other parts of the mouth. The area needing the graft is opened surgically and any diseased tissue is removed. The graft is placed and secured with sutures. A medicated material called a periodontal pack is placed over the area to protect it from contamination. This material hardens and helps reduce swelling and pain. Antibiotics are usually given after gum grafting, and ice is recommended to reduce swelling and pain. In about a week, the pack and sutures are removed.

Scraping of plaque and calculus—hardened deposits of mineral salts—at the bottom of gum pockets is called *curettage*. Local anesthesia is administered on one quarter of the mouth (e.g., the lower right) and damaged and inflamed tissue as well as plaque and calculus are removed from the roots of the teeth and the walls of the gum pockets. Different sized spoon-shaped instruments called curettes are used for this procedure.

After gum surgery, it is very important to practice good oral hygiene at home, or infections and the original problem will recur. A soft diet is usually recommended directly after surgery.

For more information on gum problems, see Gum Disease; and Gums, Receding in Part Two.

Implants

An implant is an extension of a tooth root or the replacement of a tooth by insertion of a post into the upper or lower dental ridges. This post serves to support the tooth crown or dentures. Implants are alternatives to fixed bridges and removable partial and full dentures. Some individuals do not like the acrylic and metals used for full and partial dentures. These prosthodontics may feel bulky and interfere with taste sensation and position of the tongue since they cover the roof of the mouth. Speech may also be altered. In addition, fixed bridges must be attached to teeth adjacent to spaces left by missing teeth. One big advantage of implants is that no adjacent teeth are required for attachment.

There are three types of implants—subperiosteal, endosseous, and osseointegrated. The procedure for the *subperiosteal implant* consists of surgically opening the gum and the periosteum (tissue directly under the gums and over the bone) over the area of the missing tooth or teeth. A mold or impression is taken of the area and the gums are sutured back. A metal implant, usually made of chrome-cobalt metal and containing attachments for teeth, is constructed. The area is surgically opened again, and the implant is either fastened to or allowed to sit on the bone. The gums are sutured once again. Eventually, tissue forms around the implant, holding it in place. Crowns or permanent dentures are then fastened to the attachments protruding from the implant. The disadvantages of this type of implant include the possibility of infection around the implant and its eventual failure. Even if no infections occur, the subperiosteal implants become loose over time. Implants made for the lower jaw last up to ten years, and those made for the upper jaw last up to five years. After that point, they should be removed surgically.

Endosseous implants are placed inside bone. Holes are drilled in the bone, and either wedge-shaped blades or cylinder-shaped screws are placed in the bone. The blades and cylinders, made of chrome-cobalt metal, have attachments for permanent dentures or crowns. The disadvantage of this form of implant is that the drilling may cause overheating and friction in the bone where the implant is to be inserted. This heated bone may not provide adequate stability for the implant, causing it to become loose over time. Infections are also a possibility with endosseous implants. If the infection is severe enough, the implant and the bone and gums around it have to be removed. After this, it is impossible to accommodate a new implant or a fixed or removable prosthesis.

Osseointegrated implants were first developed in the 1960s. This form of implant is made of titanium instead of chrome-cobalt metal. Titanium has been found to be better tolerated by the body's tissues. It is also very stable because it allows bone tissue to grow around it. In fact, an osseointegrated implant becomes stronger over time, as the bone thickens and becomes more attached to it. Titanium cylinder implants are the most popular of the implants; they appear to have the least risk, they become stronger over time, and they cause minimal bone resorption (if any). They also feel and function like natural teeth.

All implants must be performed by an oral surgeon or periodontist, or by a general dentist with proper training and experience in implant surgery. Implant surgery is a two-step procedure. Initially, you are evaluated using a variety of techniques including Panorex, tomograms, or cephalometric x-rays (see X-Ray Techniques in Part Three). The procedure is performed in the dentist's office, usually under local anesthesia; however, the operating environment must be equipped as a hospital and hospital sterilization standards must be followed.

First, an incision is made through the gum where the implant is to be inserted. Using sterile water as cooling irrigation, the dentist slowly drills holes into the bone. The cylinder anchor is inserted and slowly screwed in place. A temporary cap is placed over the opening above the anchor, and the gum tissue is sutured back in place.

To allow proper healing and to ensure that no contamination or infection takes place, the area is left undisturbed for six to twelve months. A soft diet should be followed for several weeks, and dentures or bridges should not be worn over the area. Antibiotics will be prescribed for a week or two, and a mild medication such as Tylenol may be suggested for pain control. Usually the stitches are removed within two weeks.

During the second step of this procedure, local anesthetic is administered and a small incision or cut is made over the implant area. The protective cap is removed and abutment cylinders are inserted in the anchored implant. These abutments extend slightly above the gums and will be ready to receive the bridge or dentures about two weeks later. After the abutments are inserted, the gums are sutured back.

Once complete healing has taken place, the denture or crown to be attached to the implant is made. Impressions are taken using the same techniques used to make standard bridges or dentures, and these impressions are sent to a laboratory for fabrication. When completed, the dentures or crowns are fastened to the implant. They remain in place, unless the dentist removes them for periodic cleanings.

For more information on surgical guidelines, see Surgery in Part Three.

Occlusal Therapy

See Equilibration.

Oral Hygiene

The practice of proper oral hygiene is the most important thing you can do for your teeth and gums. In Part One, you learned that brushing alone is not sufficient to care for your teeth. In addition to brushing, your daily routine should include flossing and, depending on your particular need, the use of balsa-wood toothpicks, gum stimulators, or water-irrigating devices.

BRUSHING

Proper brushing involves choosing and caring for your toothbrush as well as using it correctly. There are many different types of toothbrushes available, with a variety of sizes, shapes, and lengths. No single type is best for everyone, but soft bristles are recommended whether you use an electric or manual toothbrush.

Although electric toothbrushes are effective in plaque removal and gum stimulation, they have no proven advantage over manual toothbrushes. Some people, however, simply prefer them. Handicapped individuals, those who wear braces, and lazy children may also benefit from using electric toothbrushes. (For more information on electric toothbrushes, see margin copy on page 102.)

If you use a manual toothbrush, choose one with a handle that is easy to manipulate. Small-headed brushes are preferable since they have better access to all areas of the mouth. Nylon and natural bristles are equally satisfactory, but natural bristles may not last as long as nylon. Toothbrushes should be replaced every month and whenever the bristles begin to bend or fray. It is also very important to change toothbrushes after recovering from a cold or other respiratory infection since the bristles may harbor the harmful organisms.

Kept in a moisture-rich environment such as a bathroom, toothbrushes tend to harbor bacteria. Store your toothbrush in a solution of hydrogen peroxide or rubbing alcohol. Replace the solution when it begins to appear cloudy.

Now that you know how to care for your toothbrush, turn your attention to proper brushing technique. How thorough you are in your brushing is more important than how hard you brush. Follow a specific brushing sequence as shown in Figure 3.10. Begin by brushing the outside surfaces (cheek and lip side) of the upper, then the lower teeth. Start with the back teeth on one side and work your way around to the other side. Next, brush the inner surfaces of first the upper teeth, then the lower teeth. Finally brush the chewing surfaces. The key is to take your time. It is more important to brush thoroughly once a day than to brush quickly and haphazardly three or four times a day. Take at least three minutes to brush your teeth. Brush so that you are cleaning every side of every tooth: outside (cheek side), inside (tongue or palate side), and chewing surfaces.

There are three acceptable brushing methods as illustrated in Figure 3.11; but, no matter which technique you use, as stated earlier, the key is how thorough you are, not how hard or how many times you brush. All of the following brushing techniques are acceptable:

- Place the head of the brush at a 45-degree angle to the length of the tooth. Gently vibrate the toothbrush at the gum line and on the surfaces of each tooth.
- Place the brush at the gum line and roll or sweep it towards the top surface of the tooth.
- Rotate the brush in a circular motion on the gum line and the tooth surface.

In all of the above methods, the gums as well as the tongue should also be brushed as they harbor bacteria.

FLOSSING

Plaque build-up, which can lead to tooth decay and gum disease, cannot be removed from teeth by brushing alone.

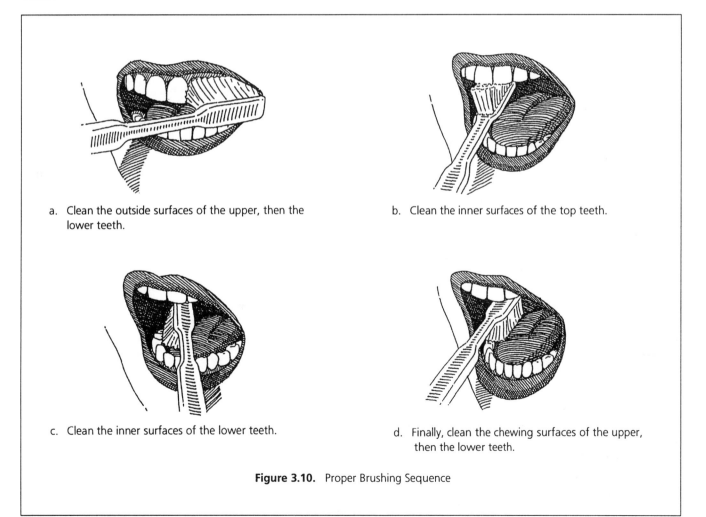

a. Clean the outside surfaces of the upper, then the lower teeth.

b. Clean the inner surfaces of the top teeth.

c. Clean the inner surfaces of the lower teeth.

d. Finally, clean the chewing surfaces of the upper, then the lower teeth.

Figure 3.10. Proper Brushing Sequence

179

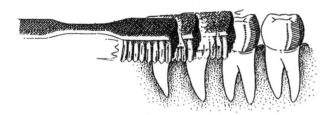

Vibrating Motion
Hold the brush at a 45-degree angle to the length of the tooth and vibrate it at the gum line and on tooth surfaces.

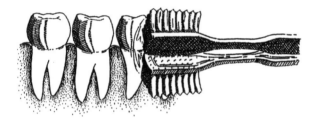

Sweeping Motion
Place brush at the gum line and sweep or roll it toward the top of the teeth.

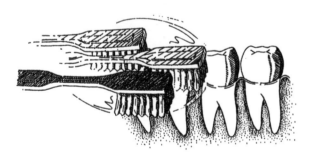

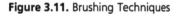

Circular Motion
Rotate the brush in a circular motion from the gum line around the tooth surface.

Figure 3.11. Brushing Techniques

Regular flossing cleans away plaque and food particles from those areas between teeth that the toothbrush cannot reach. Flossing is also an important tool for preventing gum disease. However, if the gums between the teeth have become flat, are severely receded, or have formed deep pockets, flossing will not be effective.

Several types of dental floss are available. Unwaxed floss is thinner than waxed and is best for getting into tight areas; however, unwaxed floss does fray more easily than waxed. Although the unwaxed variety is more effective in removing plaque, waxed floss is easier to handle if rough fillings are present or if teeth are very close together. Waxed floss also comes in a variety of flavors. Dental tape is a flat, wide floss that is used in areas where large spaces exist between teeth. Johnson & Johnson makes good quality floss.

To get the most out of flossing, use the following proper technique:

1. Hold approximately one inch of floss taughtly between two fingers as shown in Figure 3.12. (Holding more than one inch between the fingers will result in less control.)

2. To clean the teeth, slowly and gently, move the floss in an up-and-down and back-and-forth motion, as seen in Figure 3.13.

3. To clean the gums, curve the floss around the base of the tooth. Gently move the floss back and forth under the gums.

4. To remove the floss, use the same back-and-forth motion to bring the floss up and away from the teeth. Never force or snap the floss (either when putting it in or taking it out). This motion may cut or bruise delicate gum tissue.

A floss threader, shown in Figure 3.14, is helpful for cleaning under a fixed bridge. And if you do not have the manual dexterity to hold the floss properly with your fingers, try using a floss holder, seen in Figure 3.15.

It is important to floss daily, and only once a day is necessary (before brushing at bedtime is recommended). It may also be necessary to floss at other times throughout the day to remove food that may have gotten trapped between teeth.

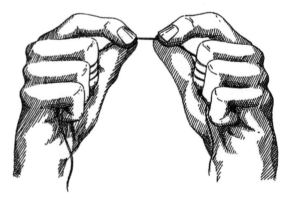

Figure 3.12. Holding Floss

USING GUM STIMULATORS

Rubber-tipped stimulators, seen in Figure 3.15, are used to massage gums and improve circulation. The rubber tip is conical and sometimes attached to the end of a toothbrush. There is some controversy regarding the benefits of these stimulators. Some dentists feel that overstimulating the gums will cause them to thicken. They also believe that some patients falsely put too much confidence in the stimulators, and don't spend enough time flossing and brushing. Other dentists feel that after gum surgery, rubber-tipped stimulators do help promote healing by their massaging action. The tips are actually best used to massage gum areas in the spaces between teeth or in the molar (back teeth) area where the gums have receded and the roots are exposed.

To use the stimulator correctly, gently place the tip against the side of the tooth at a 45-degree angle. Using a vibrating motion, press the tip against the gum area.

USING PROXI-BRUSHES

Proxi-brushes, seen in Figure 3.15, are very small, cone-shaped brushes that resemble miniature pipe cleaners. They are used to clean between exposed roots of back teeth and deep gum pockets. These brushes, which are secured to the end of a handle, are placed against the side of the tooth or between exposed roots of back teeth

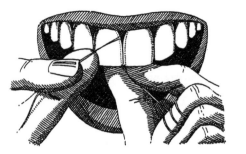

Gently slide floss between teeth.

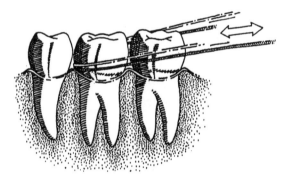

Move floss back and forth.

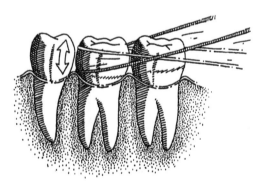

Move floss up and down.

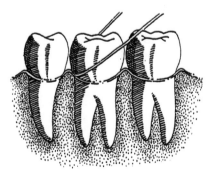

Move floss under gums.

Figure 3.13. Proper Flossing Technique

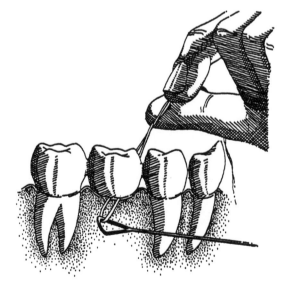

Figure 3.14. Flossing Under Fixed Bridge
with Floss Threader

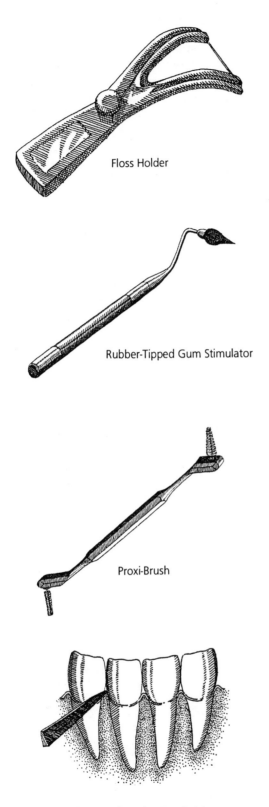

Floss Holder

Rubber-Tipped Gum Stimulator

Proxi-Brush

Balsa-Wood Wedge Toothpick

Figure 3.15. Oral Hygiene Devices

and are moved back and forth, in and out. When deep pockets are present due to gum disease, the thinnest of these tapered brushes is placed very gently in the gum pocket to clean the area.

USING TOOTHPICKS

In addition to proxi-brushes, toothpicks and wooden wedges are used to clean areas between spacy teeth and between exposed roots of back teeth. They are also beneficial for cleaning under bridges. If toothpicks are used forcibly and on a daily basis, they may wear the sides of the teeth causing "toothpick abrasion."

When the gums have receded, balsa-wood wedge toothpicks, shown in Figure 3.15, are used to clean the area between the gum and the tooth. The toothpick is first softened by moistening it in the mouth. It is then pressed firmly against the side of the tooth and gently moved in and out between the teeth.

USING WATER-IRRIGATING DEVICES

Water-irrigating devices use water under pressure to flush out debris between and around teeth. Used properly, these devices can help keep teeth clean and gums healthy. Water-irrigating devices should not take the place of brushing and flossing, but may be used as a beneficial part of your oral hygiene regimen (especially if you tend to accumulate large amounts of plaque). They also work well for those with braces.

Because water pressure from such a device may cause bacteria and debris to move under the gums or into gum pockets, it is advisable to get a deep cleaning by a dentist, hygienist, or periodontist before using one. It is also important to use the device at its low or medium setting only, never the high setting. If the water pressure is too great or the tip of the irrigator is placed incorrectly, delicate gum tissues can be damaged. Furthermore, if deep gum pockets are present, high water pressure may cause debris or bacteria to move deeper under the gums. Carefully follow directions that come with the irrigator.

Orthodontic Techniques

Abnormalities in the development of the jawbone as well as poor oral habits, trauma, and injury may cause crowding of teeth and bad bite (malocclusion). When teeth are not in their proper relationship to each other due to any of these causes, orthodontic treatment is indicated. The severity of the imbalance will determine which corrective orthodontic approach is likely to be the most effective.

If the jaw is too small to accommodate all the teeth, certain teeth may be extracted to make room. After extraction, if any of the remaining teeth are rotated (crooked), an appliance may be placed to correct the rotation. Appliances are also used to correct cross-bite, a condition in which the lower teeth overlap the upper teeth. More severe imbalances are corrected with braces as well as a "headgear," which is used to reposition the jaw. And in some instances, surgery is the only means by which the position of the jaw may be corrected.

Orthodontists utilize many different types of appliances, which may be either fixed or removable, to help move teeth, retrain muscles, and directly affect the growth of the jaws. These appliances place gentle pressure on the teeth and jaws. Braces or appliances are adjusted monthly to bring about the desired results, which may be achieved within a few months to a few years.

FIXED APPLIANCES

Braces, shown in Figure 3.16, are the most common

fixed (not removable) appliances used to correct severe tooth misalignments; they are held in the mouth with bands, wires, and brackets. Bands are first attached to all of the teeth or to selected teeth, which are used as anchors for the appliance. Wedge-shaped spacers are sometimes placed between the teeth to open areas for the bands to be inserted. Brackets are bonded to the teeth, either on the outside or, if aesthetics is a concern, on the tongue side of the teeth. The brackets may be made of metal, or clear or tooth-colored plastic. Archwires are then passed through the brackets and extended to the bands. One or more archwires may be used. The ends of the wires pass through small tubes that are attached to the bands. Elastic loops called ligatures are used to bind the wire to the brackets and to protect them during chewing. Small rubber bands may be used to hook on the bands or the wire. These are removed while eating.

Under certain conditions, a headgear may be used to provide traction. With this device, a strap is placed around the head or neck to which a face bow is attached, as seen in Figure 3.17. Headgear slows the growth of the upper jaw. It also serves as an anchor to hold the back teeth where they are, while the front teeth are pulled back.

Special fixed appliances may also be made for habit control. Attached to the teeth by means of bands, these applicances control thumb-sucking or tongue-thrusting. Because they are very uncomfortable during meals, such appliances should be used only as a last resort.

If a baby tooth is lost prematurely, a fixed appliance called a space maintainer, seen in Figure 3.16, is made to keep the space open until the permanent tooth

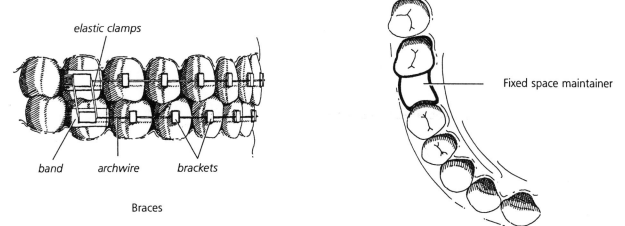

elastic clamps

band   archwire   brackets

Braces

Fixed space maintainer

Figure 3.16. Fixed Orthodontic Appliances

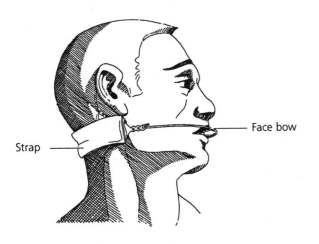

Figure 3.17. Head Gear

erupts. A crown or band is cemented over the tooth that is adjacent to the space, and a wire is extended from this band or crown to the tooth that is adjacent to the other side of the space. The bands and wires are placed on an acrylic base.

REMOVABLE APPLIANCES

Removable appliances can be taken out of the mouth and replaced at will. As a result, they may be easily lost or misplaced. Moreover, these applicances may not be worn as often as they should be, which prolongs the time needed to produce results. Most removable appliances should be worn all the time except while eating.

Some appliances are worn for limited times, such as at night only.

One type of removable appliance is the palatal expander—a device used to widen the arch of the upper jaw. It is a plastic plate that fits over the roof of the mouth. Outward pressure is applied to the plate by screws that force the sutures or joints in the bones of the palate to open lengthwise.

Removable appliances can also be used to bring about minor movement in the position of teeth. Some appliances are used to open spaces between teeth to make room for teeth that have not erupted. Other devices include removable jaw-repositioners, lip and cheek bumpers, space maintainers, and retainers.

Jaw-repositioning appliances are made of acrylic. Worn on either the top or lower jaw, they may cover some or all of the teeth. They are used to influence the jaws to close in a more favorable position. Also called splints, these appliances may be used for temporomandibular joint disorders.

Lip and cheek bumpers are designed to keep the lips or cheeks away from the teeth. Lip and cheek muscles can exert pressure on the teeth, and these bumpers help relieve that pressure. Bands are placed on the molars and the removable wire bumper is attached to the band as seen in Figure 3.18.

Removable space maintainers serve the same function as fixed space maintainers. The removable appliances are made with an acrylic base that fits over the jaw, and have plastic or wire branches between specific teeth to help keep the space between them open, as seen in Figure 3.18.

After completion of orthodontic treatment, a remov-

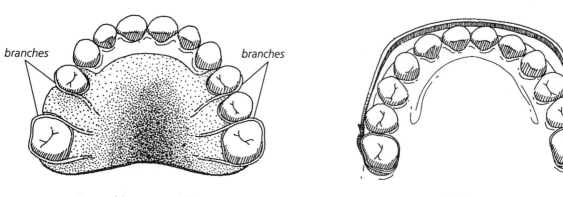

Removable space maintainer

Lip bumper

Figure 3.18. Removable Orthodontic Appliances

able retainer is worn to prevent shifting of the teeth to their previous position. The most common type is the Hawley retainer. Like most of the other removable appliances, the Hawley is made of an acrylic base and, depending on its use, may require bands on the molars and wires around certain teeth. In addition to preventing teeth from shifting, this retainer may be modified and used to prevent thumb-sucking. The retainer, which is worn on the roof of the mouth, has wire branches extending down to the lower jaw, making it impossible for the thumb or other fingers to get into the mouth.

Periodontal Techniques

See Gum Surgery.

Prosthodontic Techniques

The word *prosthodontics* is derived from Greek and means "artificial replacements for teeth." However, the prosthodontist repairs as well as replaces teeth. Prosthodontic techniques include repair of damaged teeth with crowns or onlays, replacement of one or a few missing teeth with a bridge, replacement of many missing teeth with a removable partial or a complete denture, and stabilization of loose teeth with a splint.

CROWNS

When damage to a tooth covers a considerable area, a filling may not be enough to restore it. In this case, the enamel is often replaced with a cap or crown, as shown in Figure 3.19.

First, an impression of the tooth that needs the crown must be made. Local anesthesic is administered, then the dentist removes the enamel and some of the dentin from the tooth with a drill. Usually, two to three millimeters of tooth structure is removed. A retraction cord

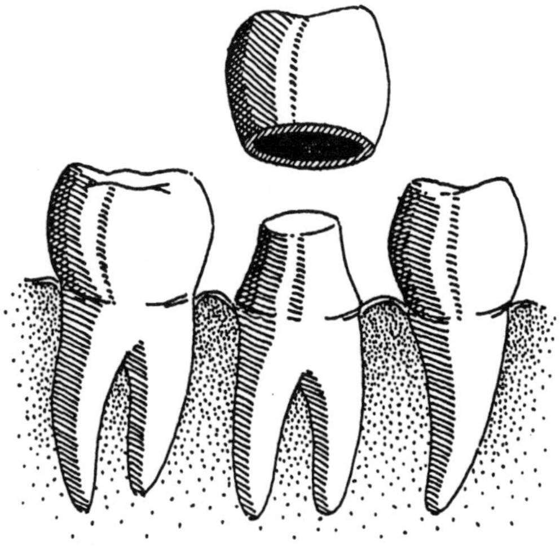

Figure 3.19. Crown

is packed under the gums to push them back from the teeth, which prevents the impression from becoming contaminated by blood and saliva. Pushing the gums back also allows the area under the gum line to be visible, insuring an accurate impression. Impressions are taken of both the prepared tooth and the opposing teeth. These two impressions and an impression of the biting surfaces of the teeth as the jaws close allow the laboratory to duplicate the relationship of the teeth as they come together in a bite.

The dental laboratory makes cast models from the impressions, mounts them on an articulator as shown in Figure 3.20, and fabricates the crown based on the dentist's instructions regarding the material to be used. Although crowns can be made of gold or other metals, porcelain crowns are aesthetically superior since they match the color of natural teeth and can be made in any shape or size. If porcelain is used, the dentist's prescription will also include the desired shade. Porcelain is usually baked onto a metal for added strength. On the front teeth, where excessive chewing forces are not a consideration, a porcelain jacket may be made without the underlying metal.

A temporary crown, usually made of acrylic or aluminum, is cemented on the prepared tooth, and worn until the permanent crown is placed. Usually within two weeks, the crown is ready. Before the dentist cements the new crown in place, he or she will check to make sure that it seals tightly over the prepared tooth,

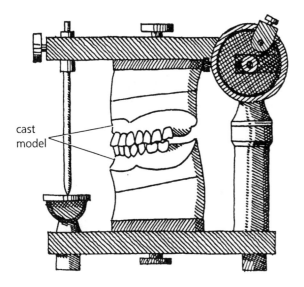

Figure 3.20. Articulator

the bite is correct and meets properly with the opposing teeth, and, if it is porcelain, the color matches well with the other teeth.

BRIDGES

Missing teeth should be replaced promptly or malocclusion (bad bite) will result. Gaps left by missing teeth eventually cause the remaining teeth to rotate or shift into the empty spaces, resulting in the bad bite. Malocclusion and the imbalance it produces increases the likelihood of gum disease and temporomandibular joint disorders (see TMJ in Part Two.) Another obvious reason to replace missing teeth is that the gaps are not aesthetically pleasing.

Bridges, of which there are a few types, are commonly used to replace one to three missing teeth. They span the space where the teeth are missing. The teeth that are located on each side of the space are called abutments; they serve as anchors for the bridge. The actual bridge refers to the false tooth (or teeth)—called a pontic—with a crown at each end. These crowns are cemented or bonded to the abutments, as seen in Figure 3.21.

Fixed Bridge

The crowns on the ends of a fixed bridge are permanently cemented to the abutment teeth. Before making a fixed bridge, first the abutment teeth are trimmed with a drill. An impression or mold is made and sent to a dental laboratory, where the bridge is then fabri-

cated. (Temporary crowns are placed on the abutments until the bridge is ready.) A fixed bridge is usually made of some type of metal (e.g. gold). For aesthetic purposes, porcelain may be baked onto (fused to) the metal.

The advantage of a fixed bridge is that it is strong and very comfortable (most people forget they are even wearing one). They are also permanent unless removed by a dentist. Occasionally, a fixed bridge may become loose from chewing on very sticky foods such as taffy.

Bonded Bridge

The bonded bridge is similar to the fixed bridge, and it is fabricated using the same procedure. The major difference is that this type of bridge is bonded rather than cemented to the abutment teeth. Bonded bridges are also made of porcelain (not porcelain fused to metal). Although bonded bridges are more natural looking than the porcelain-fused-to-metal types, they are not as strong. Chemicals and high-intensity light are used to bond the crowns of the porcelain bridge to the abutment teeth.

Removable Bridge

The removable bridge consists of a false tooth or teeth that are anchored to the adjacent teeth with metal clasps (see Figure 3.22). Very little trimming is done on the adjacent teeth. In order to clean the bridge, simply remove it from the mouth. One disadvantage of this type of bridge is that it is not aesthetically pleasing, since the metal clasps may be visible. Removable bridges are also less stable than fixed or bonded bridges.

Maryland Bridge

Dentists from the University of Maryland have developed the Maryland bridge, a new type of bonded bridge that requires minimal trimming of the adjacent abutment teeth. To use this bridge, the abutment teeth are trimmed slightly on the inside surface (tongue side) only. An impression of the area is then taken and sent to a dental laboratory where the bridge is fabricated. Rather than crowns, the Maryland bridge has metal wings that are bonded to the inside surfaces of the abutment teeth, as seen in Figure 3.23.

When the bridge is ready to be placed, the abutment teeth are acid-etched on the inner (tongue side) surfaces only. Using chemicals and high-intensity light, the metal wings are then bonded or "cured" to the abutment teeth. Because the wings are bonded to the inner surfaces only, they cannot be seen. Maryland bridges are

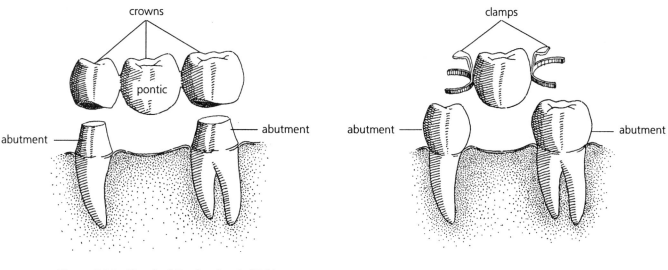

Figure 3.21. Standard Fixed or Bonded Bridge

Figure 3.22. Removable Bridge

suitable for front teeth that have no cavities, cracks, or other problems on the adjacent teeth. The disadvantage of the Maryland bridge is that it may become loose easily and have to be rebonded.

Cantilever Bridge

The pontic or false tooth of a cantilever bridge is attached to the crown of an abutment tooth on one side only, as seen in Figure 3.24. This type of bridge is used when there are no teeth behind a missing tooth. For added strength, two abutments on one end are usually used. The cantilever bridge is not as strong or stable as a standard bridge, which has abutments on both ends

of the pontic. Cantilever bridges are fabricated and adhered using the same technique used with a fixed bridge.

DENTURES, FULL

In severe cases of dental decay or gum disease in which most of the teeth are affected, the dentist may remove all the teeth and replace them with artificial ones in the form of a full denture. Dentures are custom-made in laboratories from impressions taken of the patient's mouth. In most cases, the teeth are made of plastic and are attached to a pink acrylic base that fits over the dental ridge after the teeth have been removed. In the

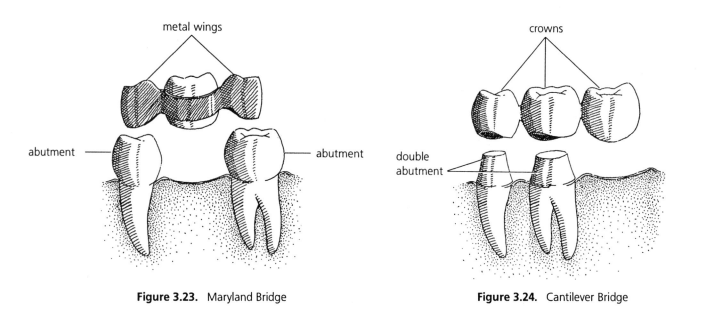

Figure 3.23. Maryland Bridge

Figure 3.24. Cantilever Bridge

upper jaw, the base also covers the roof of the mouth. Full dentures are supported by the gums and bone tissue of the dental ridge. The upper denture has the added suction of the palate, as it is made to cover this area. The lower denture does not have this added advantage because of the need to accommodate the tongue. As a result, the lower denture usually does not fit as tightly as the upper one.

The full denture is less stable than the partial denture since there are no natural teeth present for support. Chewing pressure provided by a full denture is limited compared with natural teeth, and taste may also be altered since the entire palate is covered by plastic.

The procedure for making full dentures is similar to that for making partial dentures. If teeth in the front of the mouth need to be extracted and the person does not want to wait for healing to take place before making the denture, an immediate denture may be made.

The immediate denture requires two to three dental visits. During the first visit, if any back teeth require extraction, they are pulled and the area is allowed to heal (usually two weeks). At the next appointment, impressions are taken and sent to the laboratory with specifications regarding color, shape, and size of the desired teeth. When the laboratory returns the completed denture, the dentist pulls any remaining front teeth and inserts the immediate denture. Since the gum tissue in the front will begin to heal after the denture is inserted, the base may have to be remade after a period of time. The procedure of remaking the base of the denture is called a reline.

Sometimes, the dentist may choose to leave selected roots of teeth in the bone to prevent resorption of underlying bone. The crowns of the teeth are ground down to the gum line, root canal therapy is performed on the roots, and dentures are made. These are overdentures, which rest on the tooth roots. The roots can also be used as anchors for various devices that connect the denture and improve stability. These attachments may include posts, magnets, and bars placed in the roots and underneath the denture. The disadvantage of the overdenture is that the roots may decay or cause infection and gum disease, requiring them to be pulled and new dentures to be made. Overdentures are also more difficult to keep clean compared with standard dentures.

DENTURES, PARTIAL

When several teeth are missing or when money is a consideration, a partial denture is an option. Partial dentures are less expensive than bridges; they are not fixed in place with cement, but can be removed at will.

The artificial teeth on this type of denture rest upon a metal or acrylic framework that is attached to natural teeth with clasps or rests. Metal frameworks are made of chrome-cobalt or gold; they are heavier than the all-acrylic or plastic frames. Whether teeth are missing on one or both sides of the mouth, most frameworks are horseshoe-shaped and extend to both sides for support. In the lower jaw, the framework is extended in a way that allows movement of the tongue. In the upper jaw, it may cover the palate.

One type of partial denture, called a Nesbit, consists of an artificial tooth with clasps on either side that are fastened to adjacent teeth. The Nesbit does not extend to both sides of the mouth and is less bulky than conventional partial dentures. However, this type of denture may become loose and can be easily swallowed. Most people change to a standard partial denture after having a Nesbit.

One disadvantage of most partial dentures is the unsightly appearance of the metal clasps that wrap around the natural teeth. As an alternative, some partials are made with precision attachments, which are aesthetically superior to those made with metal clasps. To make precision attachments, crowns with special slots are put on teeth adjacent to the partial denture. Extensions made on the denture fit into the slots like a key. When the denture is placed in the mouth, the extensions snap into the slots and hold the partial in place. Although partials with precision attachments are aesthetically superior to those with metal clamps, they are also more expensive.

Before beginning the procedure for making a partial denture, your teeth should be professionally cleaned. The dentist must check the condition of the teeth, especially ones that will hold clasps or precision attachments. All required fillings, crowns, and extractions must be completed prior to the making of a partial denture.

Once the condition of the mouth is ready, impressions are taken of both jaws, from which study models are made. The dentist usually shows these models to the patient, and discusses how the partial denture will look and fit. During the next visit, the teeth requiring clamps, rests, or precision attachments are prepared, and a final impression is taken and sent to the laboratory. The laboratory makes the framework and sends it back to the patient for a fitting. Once this is done, teeth for the denture are selected for color and size, and the framework is once again sent to the laboratory. The patient then has another opportunity to try the framework, only this time with the teeth placed in wax. If the appearance and fit of the denture is satisfactory, it is returned to the lab for completion. During the final office visit, the dentist inserts the partial denture in the mouth and and gives the patient instructions on proper care and use. (For more information, see Denture-Related Problems in Part Two.)

ONLAYS

Teeth that are damaged severely by decay or wear but have enough tooth structure not to warrant a crown are restored with an onlay. Since onlays are made to restore back teeth that must withstand chewing pressure, gold is the material of choice. When aesthetics is a concern, a porcelain onlay may be made. The porcelain onlay will match natural teeth, but may fracture because it does not have the added strength of metal.

The procedure used to make onlays is similar to that used to make crowns: the tooth is prepared with a drill, impressions are taken, a temporary onlay is placed, and the final onlay is inserted and cemented in place at a subsequent office visit.

SPLINTS

If teeth become slightly loose but are otherwise healthy, they may be stabilized with splints. A splint binds a loose tooth firmly to adjacent teeth, preventing it from becoming looser. The dentist uses a drill to make troughs, usually on the tongue side of the teeth. A nylon string or wire is laid into the trough, which is filled with tooth-colored composite. The procedure is completed in one office visit. Once the loose tooth appears to have stabilized, the wire or nylon string is removed and the troughs are filled with composite.

Root Canal Therapy

See Endodontic Problems in Part Two; and Endodontic Techniques in Part Three.

Sealant Application

If a dentist told you there was a way to protect your teeth so that you would never get cavities, would you be interested? Sealants are a good way to prevent cavities from starting.

In children, cavities are most likely to occur on the chewing surfaces of back teeth (on baby teeth as well as permanent teeth). These surfaces have pits and grooves that are easily missed during brushing and, therefore, collect bacteria that cause cavities. Sealants, which are made of resins, cover and protect these areas. Although sealants are used on baby teeth as well as permanent teeth, they are more commonly used on newly erupted permanent molars.

The technique for applying sealants is very similar to that used to bond cosmetic filling materials. Phosphoric acid in a concentration of 30 to 50 percent is applied to the chewing surfaces of the molars. The acid is left on the tooth for a minute to etch the surface. Acid-etching is necessary for good adhesion of the sealant to the tooth. Next, the sealant is painted onto the tooth. A visible blue light is used to harden this material in place. The resin forms a hard covering over the grooves and pits in the tooth, preventing bacteria from producing cavities.

If applied properly, the seal should last a minimum of two years, and may be reapplied when it wears away. It is very important that the area be kept dry while applying the sealant, or contamination from saliva will be sealed in the area. Before the sealant is applied, it is also important for the tooth to be thoroughly cleaned and free from decay. If any signs of decay are ignored and the tooth is sealed, the decay will spread rapidly under the seal.

The cost of sealants varies, depending on the dentist. The usual cost is about $25 to $35 per tooth. Most insurance carriers do not cover the cost of sealants.

Stress and Anxiety Management

Anxiety and physical tension go hand in hand. By using some simple relaxation techniques, you can greatly reduce your physical tension and, in turn, reduce any anxiety you may feel. These self-help techniques can be used both before the office visit and during the visit to increase your level of comfort. When necessary, your doctor or dentist can also provide medication to reduce your anxiety.

USE RELAXATION TECHNIQUES

One simple exercise to help you become physically relaxed involves concentrated breathing and relaxing groups of muscles until your whole body is calm. Follow these simple steps:

1. Inhale slowly and count to four in one-second intervals. As you are counting, introduce words like "calm," "relax," "peaceful," "serene," and "tranquil" in your mind.

2. As you exhale, count to four in one-second intervals and let your face and neck muscles relax.

3. Repeat the inhalation procedure.

4. Exhale, counting to four at one-second intervals and letting your shoulder muscles relax.

5. Repeat the inhalation procedure.

6. Exhale, counting to four at one-second intervals and letting your arm and hand muscles relax.

7. Repeat the inhalation procedure.

8. Exhale, letting your stomach muscles relax, then your leg muscles, and finally your foot muscles.

Guided imagery or visualization is another method used to help combat anxiety. Instead of focusing on the treatment, paint a picture in your mind of another place. Visualize a warm, sunny day at a beach or see yourself on a mountain near a stream or a waterfall. Hear the sounds of the ocean waves, the sea gulls, and the laughter of children. Listen to the sound of the stream or the waterfall. See yourself swimming in the water and feeling wonderfully relaxed and refreshed. Get into these scenes and have fun with them. Feel warm sand between your toes as you walk on the beach. Look at the incredible flowers around you on the mountain and smell their perfume. Let your imagination take you away.

Another technique is to use the time during treatment to plan projects, meditate, or pray. Reassure yourself that you are in good hands and that you have confidence in your dentist. Learn the acupressure points (see Acupressure in Part Three), and treat yourself for anxiety and pain while you are receiving dental treatment.

HELP YOUR CHILD

During a child's first appointment, have the dentist show the child the equipment and instruments and explain what each thing does. Unless it is an emergency, the first appointment should consist of only an exami-

nation and perhaps a cleaning. Return for fillings or extractions, and prepare the child for the return visit.

Talk to the child before the appointment and be honest with him or her. Explain that there may be a little pinch if a shot is given (pinch the arm so the child will know what it may feel like). Children model themselves after their parents; if you describe how horrible and painful your experience was at the dentist's office, your child will anticipate the same.

Children who are receiving treatment—including injections of anesthesia—should be instructed to wiggle their toes one by one. Tell them they are in a contest and the best toe-wiggler wins. This diversionary tactic will help keep the child's mind off the treatment.

LEARN ABOUT DRUGS

Although it is not encouraged, tranquilizers or other relaxants may be prescribed to reduce anxiety during dental treatment. Treatment may also be rendered in conjunction with gases such as nitrous oxide, known as laughing gas; or under general anesthesia, which renders you unconscious and insensitive to pain. Due to the side effects and possible risks inherent with deep anesthetics (see Anesthesia in Part Three) and antianxiety medications, it is best to use relaxation techniques. In addition, drugs do not address the causes of the anxiety, and the medication is temporary.

Medications used for antianxiety may include small doses of diazepam (Valium) and chlordiazepoxide (Librium) taken before treatment. Barbiturates may be prescribed for their sedative action. These may include methohexital (Brevital), pentobarbital (Nembutal) and thiopental (Pentothal). Nonbarbiturate sedatives commonly used on children include chloral hydrate and glutethimide. Although usually used to diminish pain, narcotics such as meperidine (Demerol) and fentanyl (Sublimaze) may also be prescribed for their sedative action.

See also Pain and Anxiety in Part Two.

Surgery

Although most dental procedures are considered nonsurgical and can be done by general dentists, there are some more serious procedures that do require surgery. Most dentists are able to perform many minor surgical procedures, while some oral surgeries are usually left to the expertise of specialists. Dental surgery may be required for procedures that range from pulling impacted teeth to removing cancerous tumors from the mouth.

Periodontists perform surgeries that involve removal of gingival tissue due to advanced gum disease. Dental implants must be performed by periodontists, oral surgeons, or general dentists with proper training and experience in implant surgery. Surgeries involving a tooth's dental pulp and root, such as root amputations and apicoectomies, are done by endodontists. Oral surgeons are generally called upon to perform extractions of impacted teeth (usually wisdom teeth). Along with maxillofacial surgeons in a hospital setting, oral surgeons also perform operations to correct cleft lip and palate, malformed or broken facial bones, and jaw problems resulting from advanced temporomandibular joint disorders.

Specific conventional, nutritional, homeopathic, and herbal treatments are given along with the individual dental problems in Part Two of this book. See Cleft Palate and Lip; Endodontic Problems; Gum Disease; Impacted Teeth; TMJ; Tooth, Loss of; Wisdom-Teeth-Related Problems.

The following recommendations are general guidelines to consider before undergoing any surgical dental procedure. Keep in mind that any dental surgery, no matter how minor, can result in complications such as pain, infection, and uncontrolled bleeding. It is important to be aware of these possible complications and do whatever you can to prevent them.

RECOMMENDATIONS

■ You will be given specific instructions to follow after surgery. It is very important to comply with these instructions.

■ Anyone with a history of rheumatic fever, scarlet fever, heart murmur, or other diseases involving the valves of the heart, or anyone who has had cardiovascular surgery, should take antibiotics before and after surgery. These conditions make it possible for bacteria to get into the blood and cause serious infections and even death.

■ Surgery should be delayed if a person has a fever or swollen glands due to the flu or other respiratory infections. This person is likely to be infectious and to have a low physical and mental tolerance for treatment.

■ If a person is taking an anticoagulant medication such as warfarin and cannot be taken off the drug during

surgery, it is advisable to handle the procedure in a hospital since bleeding will be difficult to control. People with hemophilia also require special care, and may require hospitalization during surgical procedures to minimize and prevent complications.

■ High blood pressure should be under control before any surgery.

■ Diabetics whose disease is controlled should present no problems; however, diabetics are prone to infection, and severe anxiety may trigger shock. It may be helpful for a diabetic to drink fruit juice before surgery unless food or drink are to be withheld prior to administration of general anesthesia.

■ It is very important to provide the dentist with your complete and accurate medical history, since interactions between drugs prescribed and administered may cause serious problems. Allergies, especially those involving medications, should be listed.

■ Before undergoing surgery, try to anticipate an easy, successful operation and rapid healing. Studies have shown that the body responds to this positive state of mind, and recovery is enhanced. While you are waiting for a local anesthetic to take effect, and during the procedure, visualize a successful surgery without complications. This simple technique will make the procedure easier on you and the dentist. The more tense you are, the quicker your nervous system will be to translate any sensation into pain.

■ Whenever possible, opt for local anesthesia rather than general during dental procedures and surgeries. For more information, see Anesthesia in Part Three.

■ Insurance for dental coverage varies from one policy to another. Be sure to learn the specifics of your individual dental plan before undergoing any procedures.

■ If, for any reason, you are not comfortable with the recommendation for surgery, it is wise to get a second and even third opinion.

Tooth Extraction

Teeth are extracted for a number of reasons—they are hopelessly involved with severe gum disease, they cannot be restored, or they are nonfunctional. Sometimes teeth are extracted to accommodate an orthodontic device.

Extraction of a tooth that is impacted and surrounded

by badly infected gums (pericoronitis) can often prevent the return of the infection. Extraction may also be recommended if decay has reached deep into a tooth, or an infection has destroyed a large portion of the tooth or the surrounding bone, and root canal therapy cannot restore it. A nonfunctional tooth is often a wisdom tooth that is crooked or lies opposite a space in which another wisdom tooth has already been pulled; it is not involved in normal chewing processes.

Unless it is absolutely necessary, a tooth should never be extracted. Each tooth is dependent on every other tooth to maintain its normal position and function. After a tooth is extracted, the adjacent and opposing teeth will eventually move out of normal position and lose function. As a result, new problems may develop, possibly requiring orthodontic or prosthodontic treatment. In most cases, it is important to replace the extracted tooth as soon as possible.

PROCEDURE

The first step in extracting a tooth involves a thorough evaluation based on a review of the patient's medical history, a reading of appropriate x-rays, and a thorough examination of the tooth. X-rays reveal the length, position, and shape of the tooth and the surrounding bone. From this information, the dentist can estimate the degree of difficulty of the procedure and determine if the patient should be referred to a specialist. If the dentist determines that the procedure involves minimum difficulty, then he or she will likely decide to perform the extraction.

It is very important to first anesthetize the area before removing a tooth. The amount and type of anesthetic used depends on the tooth's location, as well as the pain tolerance and medical history of the patient. Usually for a simple extraction, once the area is anesthetized, the tooth is loosened with the help of a tool called an elevator, and then extracted with dental forceps. Other tools may also be used during or following the extraction. For example, dental files may be used to smooth and recontour the underlying bone, and curettes may be used to remove dead or infected tissue from the socket. At the end of the procedure, the dentist may or may not feel the need to close the area with a suture.

For the initial forty-five to sixty minutes following the removal of a tooth, it is critical to keep the area clean to prevent infection and to promote clot formation. Before the patient leaves the office, the dentist will have him or her bite down gently on a piece of dry, sterile gauze that is placed over the area. Home care instructions will also be given to the patient.

POSSIBLE COMPLICATIONS

Although most teeth are pulled without any problems, some extractions can be more difficult than others. For example, if a tooth is severely decayed or broken, removal may require surgery (usually performed by an oral surgeon). Often the tooth will have to be taken out in pieces. Impacted teeth are also removed surgically.

Under normal conditions following tooth removal, a certain amount of pain and discomfort is expected. Discomfort should lessen within three days to two weeks. Sometimes, however, complications occur following extraction. For instance, when a lower molar is removed, numbness of the lower jaw may result. A major nerve—the inferior alveolar—is located near the roots of these molars. If the nerve is damaged during extraction, numbness may result and can last anywhere from a few hours to days to months and even permanently.

Sometimes, a tooth is embedded in the surrounding bone in such a manner that part of the bone has to be removed in order to extract the tooth. As a result of removing the bone, the surrounding gum will likely cave in. This aesthetically unappealing complication is corrected by a surgical procedure in which artificial or freeze-dried bone is embedded in the area.

Once a tooth is pulled, other complications such as uncontrolled bleeding and infection may occur. Dry socket, another post-extraction complication, can occur as the result of improper clot formation. It is, therefore, very important to follow the instructions of your dentist or oral surgeon after any tooth extraction, even a seemingly simple one.

For specific conventional, nutritional, homeopathic, and herbal recommendations following tooth extractions see Dry Socket; Endodontic Problems; Gum Disease; Impacted Teeth; Infection; Orthodontic Problems; Tooth, Loss of; Wisdom-Teeth-Related Problems in Part Two.

Using Herbs

Herbs are plants; they have roots and stems and leaves; some have flowers and berries. Where and how an herb is grown, how it is harvested, which part is used, and whether it is used fresh or dried all contribute to the herb's effectiveness. Even the method of storage is a factor since the potency of herbs may be reduced by exposure to light. If you wish to become an herbalist, there are many books you can consult for additional information.

For the purposes of this book, you should know that herbs are available in the form of capsules, tablets, liquid beverages, powders, dried leaves, extracts, tinctures, creams, lotions, salves, and oils. In Part Two, each entry describing a disorder includes a chart of herbal treatments with directions for their use. The directions tell you whether to use tablets, powders, tinctures, etc. In some cases, you are instructed to prepare an application, tea, or mouthwash. Directions for these preparations appear below.

For more detailed information on herbs, see Herbal Therapy in Part One.

TEA PREPARATION

Warm or cold teas can be used as drinks, tonics, or mouthwashes. To prepare herbal teas, use one heaping teaspoon of herb per cup of boiling water. For stronger tea, increase the amount of herb used (one to three teaspoons is a good range). If more than one herb is being used, add one-half cup of water for each additional teaspoon of herb. Pour freshly boiled water (preferably distilled) over the herbs. Do not use aluminum pots for boiling or steeping. Cover and steep for five minutes. Strain and drink as directed in Part Two.

If a tea recommended in Part Two is prepared in a different manner, the directions for preparing that tea appear below:

Alfalfa Tea

Add 2 tablespoons of dried leaves to 2 cups of boiling water, and steep for 10 minutes. Strain and drink as directed in Part Two.

Alfalfa and Red Clover Tea

Add 1 tablespoon of each herb to 1 cup of boiling water, and steep for 10 minutes. Strain and drink as directed in Part Two.

Anise and Sage Tea

Add 2 tablespoons of each herb to 1 cup of boiling water, and steep for 10 minutes. Strain and drink as directed in Part Two.

Black Cohosh, Catnip, Red Clover, and Yellow Dock Tea

Add 2 tablespoons of each herb to 4 cups of boiling water, and steep for 10 minutes. Strain and drink as directed in Part Two.

Chamomile Tea

Add 2 tablespoons of chamomile flowers to 2 cups of boiling water, and steep for 10 minutes. Strain and drink as directed in Part Two.

Echinacea, Myrrh, and Licorice Root Tea

Add 4 tablespoons of each herb to 8 cups of boiling water, and steep for 10 minutes. Strain and drink as directed in Part Two.

Wintergreen Tea

Add 2 tablespoons of leaves to 2 cups of boiling water, and steep for 10 minutes. Strain and drink as directed in Part Two.

MOUTHWASH PREPARATION

To prepare a mouthwash, follow the directions for the appropriate tea. If a mouthwash recommended in Part Two is prepared in a different manner, the directions for preparing that rinse appear below. Allow the liquid to cool before using as a mouthwash unless a warm rinse is indicated. Keep the liquid in your mouth as long as possible, swishing it around before spitting it out.

Clove Mouthwash

Add 1 tablespoon of clove oil to 2 cups of boiling water. Cool before using.

Goldenseal Mouthwash

Add 1 tablespoon of goldenseal and 1 teaspoon of baking soda to one cup of warm water. Cool and strain before using.

Myrrh Mouthwash

Add 1 tablespoon of myrrh to 1 cup of warm water. Cool before using.

Peppermint Mouthwash

Add 1 tablespoon of peppermint oil to 2 cups of boiling water. Cool before using.

Rockrose Mouthwash

Add 1 teaspoon of rockrose to 1 cup of boiling water for 10 minutes. Cool and strain before using.

APPLICATION PREPARATION

Applications can be made from liquids or gels and can take the form of compresses, poultices, swabs, etc. These applications can be used either hot or cold. Moist heat improves circulation in the area to which it is applied and tends to relax muscles by increasing the flow of oxygen to the area. Cold applications lessen pain and reduce swelling, consequently causing the muscle to relax.

Aloe Vera Gel

Make a cut on an aloe leaf. Dip a cotton-tipped applicator in the gel that appears on the cut. Use the applicator to apply the gel as directed. Do not eat or drink for 30 minutes after application.

Compress

Prepare an herbal tea or an herbal extract or oil mixed with water. (When using a tea, allow it to cool to room temperature or use warm.) Soak a cloth in the liquid and apply it to the affected area. Leave the compress on as directed in Part Two or until you feel relief.

Essential Oil Applications

Sometimes the active property of an herb is found in the oil contained in the plant. These oils—known as volatile or essential oils—are released when the plant is crushed. Essential oils are usually obtained from mints, spices, and aromatic herbs, and are applied externally.

You can purchase essential oils in herb shops, aromatherapy stores, and some health and beauty aid stores. To prepare your own essential oils, gently mix 2 ounces of macerated herb with 1 pint of oil (olive, linseed, or almond). Bake in a 115°F to 200°F oven for thirty minutes. Let cool, strain, and store the oil in a dark bottle. You can apply the oil directly to sores as directed. A small piece of cotton can be soaked with certain oils and dabbed on areas inside the mouth.

Goldenseal Application

Mix 1 tablespoon of goldenseal powder with enough water to make a paste. Apply directly to the sore area.

Goldenseal Toothpaste

Mix 1 teaspoon of goldenseal powder with enough water to make a paste.

Ointment

An ointment is the powdered form of an herb mixed with salve. This can be purchased ready to use, or can be prepared as directed under "salve."

Poultice

A poultice consists of two layers of linen or coarse cotton cloth between which hot, moist substances are placed. Poultices are applied to an area of the body to relieve pain or inflammation and to accelerate drainage of pus.

Bring 1 cup of water to a boil. Slowly add ½ cup of powdered herb to the water while stirring constantly over low heat until a paste is formed. Cornmeal or flour may be used to help thicken the paste. Spread the hot paste on the cloth. Allow the poultice to cool; test the temperature before applying the poultice for 1 to 8 hours on a sore, inflamed, painful area.

Salve/Ointment

Mix 1 tablespoon of powdered herb with 1 teaspoon of vegetable oil and 3 ounces of beeswax. Cover the mixture and place it in direct sunlight for 3 or 4 hours, or put it in an oven at low heat for 1 hour. Strain through fine cloth or sieve and allow to cool. The mixture is ready to use when firm.

Shepherd's Purse Application

Saturate a fresh piece of gauze in cooled shepherd's purse tea. Apply directly to the wound.

X-Ray Techniques

X-rays are similar to visible light rays, yet differ in their wavelength and frequency. Due to their shorter wavelength, x-rays can penetrate solid objects. The denser the object, the less it is penetrable by rays. Because there is less penetration, a shadow of the outline of that tissue is created on the x-ray. The denser the substance, the more pronounced the shadow will be. Enamel and bone cast more of a shadow than soft tissue, such as the gums or the pulp of the tooth.

X-rays are an important part of a regular oral exam. Different types of x-rays show tooth and jaw problems that cannot be seen any other way. Early detection of tooth decay is the main reason x-rays are taken.

To minimize potential risks from x-rays, most dental offices have safety features—high speed film for limited exposure, devices to limit beam size, and precise timers for consistent exposures. Lead aprons with thyroid collars are also worn by patients while x-rays are being taken. These aprons protect the thyroid and reproductive organs from harmful rays.

Different types of x-rays are used for dental diagnoses. The periapical x-ray, which shows teeth from the bottom of the roots to the top of the crown, is used to view infections around the root surfaces or the condition of the bone. Bitewing x-rays are taken with the top teeth meeting the bottom, and show the crowns and parts of the roots of opposing teeth as they meet. These are taken for periodic checkups approximately every eighteen months. A full set of x-rays consists of sixteen to twenty-four views, including periapical and bite-wings of teeth from different angles. A full set is required at least once every three to five years.

Panoramic (Panorex) films provide a complete view of the upper and lower jaws, including the joints. The Panorex is useful for determining the health of the bone and jaw, and for diagnosing the formation of cysts. This film is used by the orthodontist to check tooth eruption, and by the oral surgeon to check the eruption of wisdom teeth.

Tomography provides a clear view of the temporo-mandibular joint area and is used to evaluate TMJ disorders. Computerized tomography (CAT scan) is more sensitive and reveals subtle details of both bone and tissue. Tomograms show small, thin "slices" of an area at a time.

Arthrography is also used to diagnose TMJ disorders. A liquid dye that shows up opaque (white) on an x-ray is injected into the joint area. From the x-ray, the dentist can evaluate displacement of the disc.

Cephalometric x-rays reveal relationships of the bones of the face. These are commonly used for diagnosis and treatment of orthodontic problems.

For more information on x-rays, see X-Ray Exposure in Part Two.

Glossary

Note: Words that appear in bold italics in definitions are defined elsewhere in this glossary.

Acid-etching—treating a tooth with a mild acid solution to make the surface rough, which allows certain bonding materials to adhere better.

Abscess—a pus–filled hole that is the result of an infection.

Abutments—teeth, roots, or *implants* used to support *dentures* or a *bridge*.

Acidophilus—a *friendly bacterium* (*Lactobacillus acidophilus*) that aids in the digestion of proteins and the detoxification of harmful substances. It is found in the human intestinal tract and in soured products such as buttermilk, yogurt, *acidophilus milk*, and cheese.

Acidophilus milk—milk that has the *friendly bacterium Lactobacillus acidophilus* added to it to aid in the digestion of proteins and to help detoxify harmful substances in the human intestinal tract.

Acute necrotizing ulcerative gingivitis. *See* Trench mouth.

AIDS (Acquired Immune Deficiency Syndrome)—a fatal disease of the immune system that alters the body's ability to defend itself. It is caused by HIV (human immunodeficiency virus), which, in turn, causes a breakdown in the body's immune system, eventually leading to overwhelming infection and/or cancer.

Alveolar osteitis—inflammation of the *alveolar process*. It is caused by infection, bone degeneration, or injury. Symptoms include swelling, tenderness, dull aching pain, and redness in the tissue surrounding the affected bone.

Alveolar process—the part of the jaw that holds the teeth.

Alveoli—microscopic air sacs in the lungs that are covered by capillaries and are involved in the exchange of carbon dioxide from the blood with oxygen from inhaled fresh air.

Alveolitis—inflammation of the *alveoli*.

Amalgam—a combination of metals, usually including silver, nickel, and mercury, used to fill cavities in teeth.

Anaerobic—relating to an organism or biological process that does not require oxygen to be sustained.

Ankyloglossia—a condition in which the membrane under the tongue is too short, limiting the movement of the tongue and impairing speech. Also called tongue-tie.

Ankylosis—the abnormal immobilization of a joint. An ankylosed tooth, for instance, occurs as the result of the abnormal hardening of the tissue that connects the tooth to its socket. This results in the abnormal positioning of the tooth.

Anterior—term referring to the front area of the mouth.

Antioxidant—a group of vitamins, including A, C, and E, that protects the body or helps the body protect itself against the corrosive effect of *free radicals* on cells.

Apex—the end of the tooth *root* (the part farthest from the chewing surface).

Apicoectomy—the surgical removal of the end (apex) of a tooth *root* after which the open end of the root is sealed with an *amalgam* or *composite resin* filling.

Apthous ulcers. *See* Canker sores.

Arthrography—examination of the interior of a joint using x-rays following the injection of a radiopaque substance.

Baby teeth. *See* Deciduous teeth.

Bacteremia—the presence of bacteria in the blood.

Bacteria, friendly. *See* Friendly bacteria.

Bad Bite. *See* Malocclusion.

Bell's palsy—paralysis of the facial nerve resulting in the permanent or temporary immobilization of the eye or the mouth on either side of the face. The cause is injury to the nerve, compression of the nerve, or an unknown infection.

Bicuspids. *See* Premolars.

Bonding—a procedure in which *composite resins* are applied to teeth in an effort to camouflage stains or to recontour misshapen teeth.

Bridge—an artificial tooth or teeth supported by one or more permanent teeth.

Bruxism—the habit of tooth-grinding, especially during sleep, that can result in loose and worn teeth, gum recession, destruction of the supportive bones of the teeth, and *temporomandibular* joint (TMJ) disorders.

Calculus—hardened deposit of mineral salts formed around the teeth. Other common places where calculi form are the kidneys and joints.

Candida—a type of yeast–like fungus (*Candida albicans*) that inhabits the intestine, genital tract, mouth, and throat. Normally, this fungus lives in healthy balance with other bacteria and yeasts in the body.

Canine teeth (cuspids)—teeth next to the *incisors* with pointed *cusps* for tearing food.

Canker sores—painful noncontagious sores that form inside the mouth and on the lips. They are small and egg-shaped, with yellow or white centers that are surrounded by reddish halos.

Cementoma—an accumulation of *cementum* at the root of a tooth.

Cementum—the bonelike connective tissue that covers the root of a tooth.

Cleft lip—a birth defect consisting of one or more splits in the upper lip. This results from the failure of the upper jaw and nasal area to close in the embryo.

Cleft palate—a birth defect in which there is a hole in the roof of the mouth. This results from the failure of the two sides of the palate to join during the development of the embryo.

Composite resins—a tooth-colored mixture of plastic resin and finely ground glass. Composites are commonly used to fill cavities in front teeth and small cavities in back teeth.

Condyle—a rounded, knoblike bump at the end of a bone to which muscles attach and join the bone to nearby bones.

Craniomandibular—relating to the part of the skull that includes the braincase (*cranium*) and the lower jawbone (*mandible*), excluding the facial bones.

Crown, artificial—a restorative tooth covering for a badly decayed or fractured tooth; usually made of porcelain or gold.

Crown natural—the visible part of a human tooth that is covered by *enamel*.

Curettage—the process of scraping material from the wall of a body cavity or other surface. It is done with a blunt or sharp instrument to remove abnormal tissue or to collect tissue for tests.

Cusp—a pointed projection located on the chewing or biting surface of a tooth.

Cuspids. *See* Canine teeth.

Deciduous teeth—first set of teeth that is eventually replaced by permanent teeth; also called baby teeth.

Dentin—material making up most of the tooth's mass. It surrounds the *pulp* and is covered by *enamel*.

Denture—a partial or complete set of removable artificial teeth.

Edema—the abnormal pooling of fluid in body tissues.

Enamel—the hard, white outer covering of a tooth.

Endodontics—branch of dentistry that deals with the diagnosis, prevention, and treatment of diseases of the dental *pulp* and the tissues at the *root apex.*

Epinephrine—a drug that narrows the blood vessels. It is used in local anesthetics for faster and longer effect. Epinephrine is also used to treat stuffy nose and extreme allergic reactions.

Extrusion—the jutting of a tooth beyond its correct position.

Free radicals—atoms that form in the body and cause damage to cells, impairing the immune system and leading to infections and various degenerative diseases. Free radicals may be formed by exposure to radiation and toxic chemicals, by overexposure to the sun's rays, or through the action of various metabolic processes, such as the use of stored fat molecules for energy.

Friendly bacteria—one-celled microorganisms that aid in the digestion of food and are necessary in the production of certain vitamins, especially the B vitamins. These bacteria also prevent the growth of undesirable microorganisms that can cause disease.

Gingivectomy—the excision of infected, diseased, or enlarged gum tissue.

Gingivitis—a condition in which the gums are red, swollen, and bleeding. Most cases result from poor oral hygiene and the build–up of *plaque* on teeth.

Glossitis—inflammation of the tongue that may develop during an infection or following a burn, bite, or other injury.

Gutta-percha—the solid, rubbery sap of various tropical trees used to temporarily seal prepared tooth cavities or to fill a root canal.

Impaction, bony—a condition in which a tooth is unable to erupt normally because it is positioned against a bone.

Impaction, gingival—a condition in which a tooth is unable to erupt normally because it is positioned against the gum.

Implant, dental—the extension of a tooth *root* or the replacement of a tooth by the insertion of a *post* into the dental ridge. The *post* supports the tooth *crown*.

Implant, endosseous—an *implant* placed inside bone.

Implant, osseointegrated—an *implant* so firmly attached to bone that it appears to be part of the bone.

Incisors—the four sharp, chisel-shaped front teeth used for cutting food.

Intravenous infusion (I.V.)—a sterile fluid injected into a vein for the purpose of medication, nutrition, or hydration.

International Unit (I.U.)—a unit of measure created by a League of Nations committee to measure vitamins A, C, and E, and selenium by biological activity as opposed to weight.

I.U. *See* International unit.

I.V. *See* Intravenous infusion.

Kefir—a beverage made of cow's milk that is fermented by means of kefir grains. It is slightly effervescent and of low alcoholic content.

Laughing gas. *See* Nitrous oxide.

Maceration—the process of softening a solid by soaking it in a liquid.

Malocclusion—abnormal contact of the upper set of teeth with the lower set of teeth. Also called "bad bite."

Mandible—the lower jawbone.

Mastication—the process of chewing food.

Maxilla—the upper jawbone.

Maxillofacial—relating to the lower half of the face.

Meridians—channels of energy that are used in traditional Chinese medicine to measure the "life force" flowing to all parts of the body.

Molars—teeth in the back of the mouth with several *cusps* used for grinding food. The furthest (third) set of molars in the back of the mouth are also known as wisdom teeth.

Mucocele—a mucous tumor or an enlarged tear-secreting sac.

Nitrous oxide—a gas used as an anesthetic in dentistry, surgery, and childbirth; also known as laughing gas.

Odontoblast—one of a layer of long cells lining the *pulp* cavity of a tooth. It is capable of internal repair of the *dentin*.

Orthodontics—branch of dentistry that deals with the diagnosis and treatment of crooked or poorly aligned teeth.

Osteoblast—a cell that begins in the embryo and, during the early growth of the skeleton, aids in forming bone tissue.

Osteopath—a medical practitioner who uses conventional medical, surgical, pharmacological, and other therapeutic procedures; but looks more at the link between the organs and the musculoskeletal system.

Otolaryngologist—a physician specializing in diseases and disorders of the ears, nose, and throat, and related parts of the head and neck.

Overbite—a vertical overlapping of the upper teeth over the lower teeth.

Papillae—small nipplelike projections on the surface of the tongue.

Partials—a prosthesis that replaces one or more, but fewer than all, of the natural teeth.

Periapical—relating to the gums and bone structure that surrounds the *roots* of teeth.

Periodontal—relating to the gums and bone structure that surrounds and supports teeth.

Periodontal pack—a surgical dressing applied to the portion of a tooth between the *crown*, the *root*, and the surrounding tissue to protect a surgical wound.

Periosteum—a fiberlike tissue that covers the bones, except at their ends. It contains the nerves and blood vessels that supply the bones.

Pharynx—the throat; a tubelike structure that includes the breathing and digestive tracts.

Plaque, dental—a thin film on the teeth made up of material in saliva containing bacteria.

Pontic—the artificial tooth of a *bridge* that replaces a natural tooth, filling the space previously occupied by the natural *crown*.

Porphyrin—a biological pigment that is thought to be involved in activating hormones from the pituitary gland.

Post—a support, usually metal, used to reinforce a tooth that has had *root canal therapy*. This post helps to support an artificial *crown*.

Posterior—term referring to the back part of the mouth.

Premolars (bicuspids)—teeth between the *canine teeth* and *molars*. Bicuspids have two *cusps* and are used for tearing and crushing food.

Prosthetic—relating to a device, such as an artificial limb or palate, designed to replace a missing part of the body.

Prosthodontics—branch of dentistry that deals with both the repair and replacement of damaged or missing teeth.

Pulp, dental—soft, spongy tissue in the center of a tooth containing blood vessels and nerves.

Pulpectomy—the complete removal of the *pulp* of a tooth.

Pulpitis—infection of the *pulp* of a tooth.

Pulpotomy—removal of a portion of the *pulp* of a tooth.

Pyorrhea—an advanced stage of *periodontal* disease (periodontitis), characterized by halitosis, painful and bleeding gums, and abscesses.

Ranula—a large saclike swelling on the floor of the mouth usually caused by a blockage of the ducts of the salivary glands.

Resorption—the dissolving away of tooth or bone structure.

Root—that part of the tooth below the *crown* and extending into the jawbone. The root contains *pulp* tissue, which is removed during *root canal therapy*.

Root canal therapy—a procedure in which *root canal* space is cleaned, shaped, and filled.

Root canals—spaces in the *roots* of teeth that contain *pulp* tissue.

Root planing—a process that leaves a smooth surface on the *root* of a tooth to which new or regenerated gum tissue may attach. The root of a tooth is "planed" after it has been scraped of damaged tissue and *tartar*.

Rotated tooth—a tooth that is crooked.

Scaling—the removal of *calculus* deposits from the teeth.

Sclerosed—hardened or stiffened.

Septicemia—a condition in which harmful bacteria and toxins from bacteria circulate in the blood.

Sodium hypochlorite—a powerful germ-killing solution used as a disinfectant, especially for water.

Sores, canker. *See* Canker sores.

Stomatognathic system—all of the structures involved in speech and the reception, chewing, and swallowing of food. This system includes the teeth, jaws, chewing muscles, and the nerves that control these structures.

Subperiosteal—relating to matter beneath the *periosteum*.

Supernumerary teeth—extra erupted or unerupted teeth.

Tachycardia—an excessively rapid heartbeat.

Tartar—a salivary deposit of calcium phosphate, calcium carbonate, and organic matter on natural or artificial teeth.

Temporal bone—one of two bones on either side of the skull above the ear.

Temporomandibular—relating to the connection between the *temporal bone* and the *mandible* (lower jawbone).

Thymocyte—a cell that originates in the thymus and is similar to a white blood cell.

Tic douloureaux—spontaneous spasm of the facial

muscles, usually occuring on the right side. The spasm normally lasts for a few seconds and is followed by additional episodes spontaneously or from stimulation of trigger zones. Also called trigeminal neuralgia.

Tinnitus—noises or unpleasant sounds in the ears, such as ringing, buzzing, roaring, or clicking that are the results of hearing impairment.

T-lymphocytes—one of two kinds of white blood cells often called "killer cells" because they secrete special compounds to destroy foreign proteins. They also help the body fight the growth and spread of cancer cells.

Tomogram—an *x-ray* of various internal layers of the head and body.

Tomography—an *x-ray* process involving the rotation of the film and *x-ray* source in opposite directions around an axis located in the area of interest. This movement blurs outside structures while maintaining sharpness in the area of interest.

Tongue-tie. *See* Ankyloglossia.

Trench mouth—an inflammation of the gums characterized by pain, foul odor, and the formation of a grey film over the diseased area. Also called Vincent's disease or acute necrotizing ulcerative gingivitis.

Trigeminal neuralgia. *See* Tic douloureaux.

Ulcers, aphthous—*See* Canker sores.

Vasoconstrictor—a chemical agent that narrows blood vessels by contracting the muscles of the vessel walls, causing blood pressure to rise.

Vasodilator—a chemical agent that widens blood vessels by relaxing the muscles of the vessel walls, causing blood pressure to drop.

Vincent's disease. *See* Trench mouth.

Wisdom teeth. *See* Molars.

Xerostomia—dryness of the mouth resulting from the lack of normal salivary secretion.

X-ray, bitewing—an x-ray that reveals the *crowns* of the upper and lower teeth and portions of their sockets on the same film.

X-ray, cephalometric—an x-ray of the head, used to decide methods of straightening teeth.

X-ray, panoramic—an x-ray that provides a complete view of the upper and lower jaws, including the joints. Both the x-ray generator and film are mounted on tracks and move around the head as a series of exposures is taken.

Dental Schools

UNITED STATES

Alabama

University of Alabama
School of Dentistry
1919 Seventh Avenue, South
Birmingham, AL 35294

California

Loma Linda University
School of Dentistry
Loma Linda, CA   92350

University of California
  at Los Angeles
School of Dentistry
Los Angeles, CA 90024

University of Southern California
School of Dentistry
925 West 34th Street
Los Angeles, CA 90007

University of California at San Francisco
School of Dentistry
707 Parnassus Avenue
San Francisco, CA 94143–0752

University of the Pacific
School of Dentistry
2155 Webster Street
San Francisco, CA 94115

Colorado

University of Colorado Medical Center
School of Dentistry
4200 East 9th Avenue, Box C–284
Denver, CO 80262

Connecticut

The University of Connecticut
School of Dental Medicine
263 Farmington Avenue
Farmington, CT   06032

District of Columbia

Howard University
College of Dentistry
600 "W" Street, NW
Washington, DC 20059

Florida

University of Florida
College of Dentistry
PO Box 100445
Gainesville, FL 32610

Georgia

Medical College of Georgia
School of Dentistry
1459 Laney Walker Boulevard
Augusta, GA   30912–0200

Illinois

Southern Illinois University
School of Dental Medicine
2800 College Avenue
Alton, IL   62002

University of Illinois at Chicago
College of Dentistry
801 South Paulina Street
Chicago, IL   60612

Northwestern University
Dental School
240 East Huron Street
Chicago, IL   60611

Indiana

Indiana University
School of Dentistry
1121 West Michigan Street
Indianapolis, IN   46202

Iowa

The University of Iowa
College of Dentistry
Dental Building
Iowa City, IA   52242

Kentucky

University of Kentucky
College of Dentistry

Albert B. Chandler Medical Center
Lexington, KY   40536–0084

University of Louisville
School of Dentistry
Health Sciences Center
Louisville, KY   40292

Louisiana

Louisiana State University
School of Dentistry
1100 Florida Avenue, Building 101
New Orleans, LA   70119

Maryland

University of Maryland
Baltimore College of Dental Surgery
666 West Baltimore Street
Baltimore, MD   21201

Massachusetts

Boston University
Goldman School of Graduate Dentistry
100 East Newton Street
Boston, MA   02118

Harvard School of Dental Medicine
188 Longwood Avenue
Boston, MA   02115

Tufts University School of Dental Medicine
1 Kneeland Street
Boston, MA   02111

Michigan

The University of Michigan
School of Dentistry
1234 Dental Building
Ann Arbor, MI   48109–1078

University of Detroit
School of Dentistry
2985 East Jefferson Avenue
Detroit, MI 48207

Minnesota

University of Minnesota
School of Dentistry
515 Southeast Delaware Street
Minneapolis, MN 55455

Mississippi

University of Mississippi
School of Dentistry—Medical Center
2500 North State Street
Jackson, MS 39216–4505

Missouri

University of Kansas City
School of Dentistry
650 East 25th Street
Kansas City, MO 64108

Nebraska

University of Nebraska Medical Center
College of Dentistry
40th and Holdrege Streets
Lincoln, NB 68583–0740

Creighton University
School of Dentistry
2500 California Street
Omaha, NB 69178

New Jersey

University of Medicine and Dentistry
  of New Jersey

New Jersey Dental School
110 Bergen Street
Newark, NJ 07103–2425

New York

State University of New York at Buffalo
School of Dental Medicine
3435 Main Street
Buffalo, NY 14214

Columbia University
School of Dental and Oral Surgery
630 West 168th Street
New York, NY 10032

New York University
College of Dentistry
345 East 24th Street
New York, NY 10010

State University of New York at Stony Brook
School of Dental Medicine
Stony Brook, NY 11794–8700

North Carolina

University of North Carolina
School of Dentistry
CB 7450 Brauer Hall
Chapel Hill, NC 27599–7450

Ohio

Case Western Reserve University
School of Dentistry
2123 Abington Road
Cleveland, OH 44106

The Ohio State University
School of Dentistry
305 West 12th Avenue
Columbus, OH 44106

Oklahoma

University of Oklahoma, Health Science Center
College of Dentistry
PO Box 26901
Oklahoma City, OK 73190

Oregon

Oregon Health Sciences University
School of Dentistry
611 Southwest Campus Drive
Portland, OR 97201–3097

Pennsylvania

Temple University
School of Dentistry
3221 North Broad Street
Philadelphia, PA 19140

University of Pennsylvania
School of Dental Medicine
4001 Spruce Street
Philadelphia, PA 19104

University of Pittsburgh
School of Dental Medicine
3501 Terrace Street
Pittsburgh, PA 15261

Puerto Rico

University of Puerto Rico
School of Dentistry
PO Box 5067
San Juan, PR 00936

South Carolina

Medical University of South Carolina
College of Dental Medicine
171 Ashley Avenue
Charleston, SC 29425

Tennessee

Meharry Medical College
School of Dentistry
1005 18th Avenue North
Nashville, TN 37208

University of Tennessee Center
  for the Health Sciences
College of Dentistry
875 Union Avenue
Memphis, TN 38163

Texas

Baylor College of Dentistry
3302 Gaston Avenue
Dallas, TX 75246

University of Texas Health Sciences Center
School of Dentistry
7703 Floyd Curl Drive
San Antonio, TX 78229

Virginia

Virginia Commonwealth University
School of Dentistry
Wood Memorial Building
521 North 11th Street
Richmond, VA 23284

Washington

University of Washington
School of Dentistry
Health Sciences Building, Section 62
Seattle, WA 98195

West Virginia

West Virginia University
School of Dentistry
The Medical Center
Morgantown, WV 26506

Wisconsin

Marquette University
School of Dentistry
604 North 16th Street
Milwaukee, WI 53233

CANADA

Alberta

University of Alberta
Faculty of Dentistry
Room 3032 Dental/Pharmacy Building
Edmonton, Alberta T6G–2N8

British Columbia

University of British Columbia
Faculty of Dentistry
2199 Westbrook Mall
Vancouver, British Columbia V6T–127

Manitoba

University of Manitoba
Faculty of Dentistry
780 Bannatyne Avenue, Room D113
Winnipeg, Manitoba R3E–0W2

Nova Scotia

Dalhousie University
Faculty of Dentistry
5981 University Avenue
Halifax, Nova Scotia B3H–3J5

Ontario

University of Toronto
Faculty of Dentistry
124 Edward Street
Toronto, Ontario M5G–1G6

University of Western Ontario
Faculty of Dentistry
1151 Richmond Street
London, Ontario N6A–5C1

Quebec

Mc Gill University
Faculty of Dentistry
3640 University Street
Montreal, Quebec M3A–2B2

Universite De Montreal
School of Dental Medicine
2900 Edward Montpetit
Montreal, Quebec H3C–3J7

Universite Laval
School of Dental Medicine
Ste-Foy, Quebec G1K–7P4

Saskatchewan

University of Saskatchewan
College of Dentistry
Health Sciences Building, Room B526
Saskatoon, Saskatchewan S7N–0W0

Professional Organizations

Academy of General Dentistry
211 East Chicago Avenue
Chicago, IL 60611

Academy of Dentistry for the Handicapped
211 East Chicago Avenue
Chicago, IL 60611

American Academy of Craniomandibular Disorders
10 Joplin Court
Lafayette, CA 94549

American Academy of Pediatric Dentistry
211 East Chicago Avenue
Chicago, IL 60611

American Academy of Periodontology
211 East Chicago Avenue
Chicago, IL 60611

American Association of Endodontists
211 East Chicago Avenue
Chicago, IL 60611

American Association of Hospital Dentists
211 East Chicago Avenue
Chicago, IL 60611

American Association of Oral and Maxillofacial Surgery
9700 Bryn Mawr Avenue
Rosemont, IL 60018

American Association of Orthodontists
460 North Lindbergh
St. Louis, MO 63141

American Dental Association
211 East Chicago Avenue
Chicago, IL 60611

American Equilibration Society
8726 North Ferris Avenue
Morton Grove, IL 60053

Federation of Prosthodontic Organizations
211 East Chicago Avenue
Chicago, IL 60611

Bibliography

Balch, James F., M.D., and Phyllis A. Balch, C.N.C. *Prescription for Nutritional Healing*. Garden City Park, NY: Avery Publishing Group, 1990.

Ballentine, R. *Diet and Nutrition*. Honesdale, PA: The Himalayan International Institute, 1982.

Davis, John, D.D.S., et al. *An Atlas of Pedodontics*. Philadelphia: W.B. Saunders Company, 1981.

Holroyd, S., et al. *Clinical Pharmacology in Dental Practice*. Washington, D.C.: The C.V. Mosby Co., 1988.

Newbrun, E. "Mechanism of Fluoride Action in Caries Prevention." In *Fluorides and Dental Caries*, ed. E. Newbrun. Springfield, IL: Charles C. Thomas, 1968.

Scheinen, A., et al. "Turku Sugar Studies. Final Report on the Effect of Sucrose, Fructose and Xylitol Diets on the Caries Incidence in Man." *Acta Odontology Scandinavia* 34 (1976):139.

Socransky, S.S. "Microbiology of Periodontal Disease—Present Status and Future Considerations." *Journal of Periodontology* 48 (1977):497.

Sonis, S., et al. *Principles and Practice of Oral Medicine*. Philadelphia: W.B. Saunders, 1984.

Taintor, Jerry F., D.D.S., and Mary Jane Taintor. *The Oral Report*. New York: Facts on File Publications, 1988.

Wilson, Roberta. *Aromatherapy for Vibrant Health & Beauty*. Garden City Park, NY: Avery Publishing Group, 1995.

Zand, Janet, L.A.C., O.M.D., Rachel Walton, R.N., and Bob Rountree, M.D. *Smart Medicine for a Healthier Child*. Garden City Park, NY: Avery Publishing Group, 1994.

Index